At home in a home

Pat Young

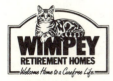

Wimpey Homes and The George Wimpey Charitable Trust offered generous financial sponsorship to allow this book to reach a wider audience than would otherwise have been possible.

A summary of Wimpey's activity in the retirement housing market can be found on page 7.

© 1988 Pat Young

Published by Age Concern England
Bernard Sunley House
60 Pitcairn Road
Mitcham Surrey CR4 3LL

Editor Margaret Adolphus
Design Eugenie Dodd
Production Joyce O'Shaughnessy
Typeset from disc by Parchment (Oxford) Ltd
Printed by Ebenezer Baylis & Son Ltd.,
Worcester

ISBN 0-86242-062-8

All rights reserved, no part of this work may be reproduced in any form by mimeograph or any other means, without permission in writing from the publisher.

Cover drawing Robin Dodd

Contents

About the author   6
About Wimpey Homes   7
Introduction   8

Chapter one
'I don't want to be a burden'   11
Facing facts
Keeping fit and active
Looking at alternatives
Stresses and strains

Chapter two
How could I go on managing at home?   19
Personal social services
Home helps · Meals-on-wheels · Lunch clubs, day centres, and day hospitals · Aids and adaptations · Other services · Finance
Health services

Chapter three
Are there any other alternatives to going into a home?   31
Moving in with the family
Sheltered accommodation
Extra-care sheltered housing

Chapter four
Are there different kinds of home to choose from? **39**

Residential care homes
Local authority homes · Voluntary homes · Private homes

Nursing homes
National health service nursing homes · Voluntary nursing homes · Private nursing homes

Homes for religious and ethnic minorities

Chapter five
How does the law protect the public? **53**

What does registration mean?
What does the Act say?
Are there any other safeguards?

Chapter six
What are my rights as a resident in a rest home? **63**

The rights of residents
Practical rights · Rules and regulations · Complaints · Privacy and autonomy · Financial affairs · If you become frail · Keeping healthy

Chapter seven
What are my rights as a resident in a nursing home? **75**

Making a good choice
Quality of care
Information · Staff · Accommodation · Complaints · Special needs · Furnishing · The patient's day ·
To sum up

Chapter eight
How do I go about finding a home?   *85*
Where?
Local authority homes
Private or voluntary homes
Your check-list
The governing factor

Chapter nine
How much will it cost, and how can I pay for it?   *95*
Local authority homes
Your financial position
Private homes
Help from the DHSS · Help from other sources · Voluntary homes · Counting the cost

Chapter ten
What will it be like and how will I cope?   *105*
Peace of mind
Someone else's experiences
A home from home

Booklist   *113*
National organisations that may help   *117*

About the author

Pat Young is a medical journalist who has edited Nursing Mirror, Geriatric Medicine, and Geriatric Nursing and Home Care. She also has wide experience of helping older people who are considering whether to go into a home.

About Wimpey Homes

Wimpey Homes, the UK's largest housebuilder, is strongly committed to the needs of the ever-increasing population of retired people.

The company currently has 20 retirement developments selling through the UK, from Bristol to Edinburgh. All are specifically designed to meet the particular requirements of elderly people, and include low-cost central heating to Electricity Council Medallion standard; full double-glazing; fully fitted and equipped kitchens; security locks to all windows and doors; easy-to-reach electric points to save bending; and wider-than-usual door frames to accommodate wheelchairs and walking frames.

All Wimpey developments are provided with a residential manager, able to respond to the 24-hour emergency alarm installed in every home. The manager also oversees the day-to-day running and maintenance of the property and surroundings and the well-being of the residents.

As a technically innovative and caring company, Wimpey is well aware of the problems faced by many retired people when deciding to leave the family home. This is reflected in Wimpey's continuing commitment to providing secure, custom-built retirement housing in the most attractive and convenient locations.

Introduction

One of the most difficult decisions we may have to make in later life is whether or not to go into 'a home'. When ill health or increasing frailty make it impossible to go on coping with the routines of daily living, the time has come to consider what the alternatives may be, and whether one should start looking for a residential home which provides the sort of care and support one needs.

Before taking such an important step, it is wise to think very carefully and to get as much information as possible on which to base your decision. This book is intended to provide such information - what different kinds of home are available, what laws and regulations govern them in order to protect the public, what to look for when you are trying to choose a home, and what the cost is likely to be. I hope it will help you to make a decision you won't regret.

Although the book is addressed directly to older people, I hope it will also be useful to the families and friends of old people, who are so often involved in this major step, or who are in a position to help and advise.

I would like to take this opportunity to express my appreciation to all those who helped me in my research, and in particular to the three residents who allowed me to interview them and quote their personal views in the final chapter. While they kindly gave permission for their real names to be used, the other names and case histories quoted are fictitious, although the circumstances described are based on fact. I have, incidentally, tried to avoid the clumsy use of 'he' or 'she' when referring to individuals, by using a single pronoun 'he' in a purely impersonal sense. No sexual discrimination is intended!

Lastly I would like to thank very warmly Mr Ralph Chapman, Principal Officer of East Sussex Social Services Department, and Miss Corrie Paxton, Chief Nurse of Eastbourne Health Authority, for reading the manuscript before publication and making many useful suggestions; and Mrs Margaret Adolphus, Head of Publishing for Age Concern England, for her unfailing patience, and encouragement.

I would like to dedicate this book to the memory of my beloved Uncle Fred (Mr F C Ross), and to my cousin Mrs Pamela Grace, a carer *par excellence.*

Pat Young
East Sussex, 1987

Chapter one
'I don't want to be a burden'

Mary Jones, a widow of 83, lived with her daughter in a small terraced house near the centre of the town in the north east of England where she and her husband had spent most of their married life. When her husband died ten years earlier, her daughter – who was unmarried – came to live with her so that she would not be alone. Mary was pleased to have someone to look after, and gladly ran the house so that her daughter Jean could carry on her job as a secretary in a local solicitor's office; and fortunately they got along very well.

In the past two or three years, however, Mary's arthritis had been getting very bad, and she found it more and more difficult to get out to do the shopping, and also to do the housework and the cooking, as her hands were getting stiff and deformed. This worried her very much, because she didn't want to become a burden to her daughter, who had given up her pleasant flat and independent life to come and live with her. The last thing she wanted was to have to ask her to give up her job as well, in order to look after the house and take care of her. And yet the doctor had told her there was no cure for arthritis, and she was bound to become more disabled by it as the years went by. Besides, her daughter couldn't afford to give up her job and a good pension when she reached retiring age.

The only alternative seemed to be for Mary to get into an old people's home – but she didn't like the idea at all of leaving her own comfortable home and treasured possessions to live in a strange place among strange people. It was extremely worrying, and Mary just didn't know what to do for the best.

Mary Jones is typical of the many older people who find that old age and ill health have combined to make it impossible for them to go on living in their own homes, either because they live alone and have no-one to look after them, or because – like Mary – they don't want to be a burden to their relatives or friends. It is an unhappy predicament to find yourself in at a time of life when all you want is to go on living, peacefully and unworried, in your own familiar surroundings and among tried and trusted friends and neighbours.

Jean, too, is typical of the many middle-aged women who have to give up their freedom and independence to care for an elderly parent or other relative who eventually becomes so dependent on them that life is reduced to an exhausting routine of washing, dressing, feeding, coping with the laundry – which may be considerable if the relative is incontinent – as well as the housework and shopping, and also trying to keep them amused or entertained. If the elderly relative becomes confused, or forgetful, or even difficult and aggressive, life for the 'carer' can be almost intolerable, particularly if there is no respite from the perpetual demands of caring.

Facing facts

Mary and Jean's story paints a gloomy picture of what can happen, but it is as well to face facts at an early stage, and to see what you can do to prevent this happening to you.

There is bound to come a time in the life of all of us who live beyond our three score years and ten when, because of increasing frailty or disability, we have to decide whether or not we can go on living at home. Unfortunately, as the years go by and we get older, our bodies – and sometimes our minds – do not function as well as they used to. Our joints get stiff, our muscles weak, and we can't get about as easily as we would like. We find it more difficult to keep our balance, and there is more risk of hurting ourselves when we fall because our bones are more brittle, and we fall more heavily because we can't save ourselves. We may not be able to hear or see as well as we could; and we may become a little forgetful or confused. All these things happen in old age as our bodies simply begin to wear out.

Besides the loss of physical and mental ability in old age, we have to be prepared to face another loss: the death of a beloved husband or wife or close friend with whom we have shared our lives. Without that person it may suddenly become impossible to carry on alone, so that we have to start looking for alternatives.

Most of us enjoy our independence, and it is not easy to come to terms with the fact that one day we may lose it. But as we get older we are able to cope more easily with problems, because we know from experience that the best way is not to hide our heads in the sand in the hope that a problem will go away, but to face up to it, get it into perspective, decide on the best way of dealing with it, and then make careful practical plans.

Advancing age has many drawbacks, but it does have one great advantage: the wisdom of experience, which we can use on our own behalf as well as to help and advise other people.

Keeping fit and active

So let's begin by facing the fact that, one day, sooner or later, we won't be able to look after ourselves any longer. What can we do to ensure that this evil day comes later rather than sooner?

First of all, don't think that every tiresome symptom you have is due to age and must be tolerated. No good doctor will say: 'What do you expect at your age?' when you complain to him of painful joints, or dizziness, or recurrent headaches.

Illness can be treated just as successfully in old age as in youth, provided that no-one – doctor, patient, or relative – regards it as inevitable.

Doctors should take more care in examining their older patients and in prescribing the right medicines in the right dosages for them because our bodies behave and react differently to drugs as we get older. This is a fact of which the medical profession has become more aware in recent years. The Royal College of Physicians has recently introduced an examination leading to a Diploma in Geriatric Medicine to enable both GPs and hospital doctors to learn more about the ageing process, how it affects the body and mind, what diseases are most likely to occur in later life, and how they can be successfully treated. This is an important step forward.

Secondly, don't think that exercise and sport are beyond you just because you are over 60 – or even that they are bad for you. On the contrary, regular exercise will do you nothing but good. It will tighten up your muscles, make your joints more mobile, tone up your heart and lungs, and even strengthen your bones. Obviously you mustn't overdo things; you must take it steadily and gently, and stop as soon as you feel tired. But it is well worth the effort to take half-an-hour's brisk walk every day, to join a keep-fit class for the over-55s, to take up golf or ballroom dancing, or to go swimming regularly. Swimming, in fact, is one of the best forms of exercise for older people, because the water supports your body-weight, but some people go on playing tennis well into their 70s, and the skiing correspondent of the Mail on Sunday is over 70 and still an active skier. But if no other form of exercise appeals to you, walking at a brisk pace in the fresh air will do you the world of good, especially if you can manage a walk daily. You will soon feel fitter and younger; the more you do the more you will be able to do, and the more you will enjoy it.

Thirdly, make sure you eat properly. Although it is true that you don't need so much food as you get older, you will still need a good balanced diet to help you to remain healthy. In particular you need plenty of vitamin C, which you get in fruit juice, freshly cooked green vegetables and salads; iron, which is contained in liver and kidneys, eggs, pulses such as beans and lentils, and dried fruit such as sultanas and raisins; fibre, which is found in wholemeal bread, high-fibre cereals like shredded wheat and porridge, wholegrain rice and pasta, digestive biscuits, and fresh fruit and vegetables; and vitamin D, which is contained in oily fish like herring, mackerel, and sardines, as well as in eggs, liver, margarine, and yoghurt. You also need to drink plenty of fluid – at least eight cupfuls a day.

So don't eat too much animal fat and sugar, but have three good meals a day – one of them hot – with fish, lean meat, or poultry and freshly cooked vegetables at your main meal, and plenty of fresh fruit and salads, wholemeal bread and pasta, and not too many biscuits and cakes. Age Concern England has published an excellent booklet called *Eating Well on a Budget*, in association with the BBC Food and Drink programme, which presents a week's menus together with some useful tips on shopping, cooking, and storing the foods which will do you nothing but good, and keep you well nourished and fit.

Older people often have trouble with their teeth, or with dentures that don't fit all that well, making eating uncomfortable, difficult, or even painful. Going for a regular dental check-up, of both your teeth and your dentures, is very important, as your dentist may be able to improve your mouth and teeth quite simply and help you to eat your food easily and without pain or discomfort.

Fourthly, take an interest in life. Our minds and bodies are very closely connected; a psychological problem is almost bound to have a physical effect, and loneliness and depression, which are understandably common in old age, can make you physically ill as well. So if you are lonely and depressed, perhaps grieving for a loved one, try to get out and about no matter how hard it is to begin with; make the effort to take up new hobbies or revive your interest in old ones; join local clubs and societies so that you get to know other people, make new friends and spend time with them. Join a class at your local adult education centre: it is never too late to learn something new.

Alan Brown, a retired accountant, lost his wife when he was 71. Lonely and unhappy, he looked round for ways of filling his time. Knowing he was interested in people, a friend suggested that he ask the Citizen's Advice Bureau in the town where he lived if they needed any voluntary helpers. He did so; they gave him a warm welcome, sent him on a training course, and now he spends one afternoon a week sorting out other people's problems and giving them helpful advice. He has always been a keen amateur singer and actor, and now he is a valued member of his church choir and of the local amateur dramatic society – and treasurer of both. He has solved his own problems by giving help, advice, and pleasure to others.

It is particularly important for a widow or widower, newly bereaved, to be able to find some comfort and support. There is an excellent organisation called CRUSE which exists to help such people: to give advice, counselling, comfort and support, and the opportunity to meet and talk to others who have gone through the same agonising experience and understand what it means to lose a life partner.

Looking at alternatives

Mary Jones might have been able to stay active a little longer if she had been conscious of the importance of diet and exercise, but her arthritis had got to the stage when it had begun to rule her life, and she had to decide what to do about it. She was torn between her longing to stay in her own home, being cared for by her loving daughter, and an overwhelming feeling of guilt about the sacrifices her daughter would have to make if she did so. She had not discussed it with her daughter because she knew she must make the decision for herself. What had not struck her was that there might be alternatives to going into a 'home' which could enable her to stay at home yet not be a burden to her daughter. The next chapter goes into these alternatives in detail.

Stresses and strains

Mary and her daughter Jean were very lucky that they got on so well together. Many families don't, and there may be all sorts of stresses and strains between different generations living together. Instead of being kind, affectionate, and considerate, Mary might have been a selfish, demanding old woman who made her daughter's life a misery. In such a situation, the daughter would be torn between her duty to look after her mother and her longing to be free of the burden. She would feel guilty and disloyal at even thinking about getting her mother into a 'home', and if she ever suggested this possibility to her mother she would be sure to have to face stormy recriminations.

It is only now being acknowledged that caring for an elderly relative can place an intolerable strain on the carer – usually a daughter, married or unmarried, who is the member of the family expected to take on this responsibility. Though they accept the role willingly and perform it conscientiously, carers need breaks from the relentless routine, and they should not feel guilty if they think they have come to the end of their tether. Finding a place for the parent in a residential care or nursing home may then be the best thing for both parties, as there will be a relief from strain on both sides and their relationship will not be stretched beyond the point of endurance. Indeed, it could be strengthened and become closer.

The boot, of course, might have been on the other foot. Mary's daughter Jean might have been the selfish, inconsiderate one, who regarded her mother as a nuisance and made no bones about showing her irritation and desire to be rid of her. Mary might be stampeded into agreeing to go into a home, or she might be only too glad to get away from her daughter. But this might mean jumping out of the frying pan into the fire. No one should allow themselves to be rushed or persuaded into going into a home against their will or better judgment. This is a recipe for disaster. The decision must be yours and yours alone, taken after a lot of careful thought and consideration. You must be as certain as you can that it is the right decision, and that you have carefully considered all possible alternatives.

Chapter two

How could I go on managing at home?

It is well known that many older people do not make use of all the services and benefits available to them, either because they just don't know what services there are, or because they are proud of being independent and don't want to be a burden to anyone. Having been responsible for themselves and their families all their lives, they are reluctant to surrender this responsibility to someone else. But they will have paid their rates and taxes all their lives, so they are entitled to what help is available from the State when they need it, and should not be hesitant – or ashamed – about seeking help. It could enable them to live independently in their own homes for a while longer, without having to rely on someone to look after them.

Personal social services

It is Government policy that older people should be enabled to live in their own homes for as long as possible when they become frail or disabled, and that services should be available to give them the support they need. This may take the form of a home help, meals-on-wheels, lunch clubs, day centres, and aids and adaptations in the home, all of which are called 'personal social services' and are supplied by the social services departments of local authorities (called social work departments in Scotland).

The quality and availability of these services varies greatly from one area to another, however. Some large private companies which up to now have confined themselves to building warden-supervised accommodation and residential care homes for the elderly are now branching out into providing the whole range of services that frail old people need. These private services are of good quality and very wide-ranging, according to the Centre for Policy on Ageing, a major research body concerned with the quality of life for older people, but usually they cost more than local authority services, which are subsidised.

Home helps

Having someone to do the household chores for you can make all the difference if, like Mary, you are becoming crippled with arthritis and find it very difficult to do them yourself. The home help service is intended to relieve elderly people of routine tasks such as housework, shopping, laundry, and preparing food. It has been calculated that each local authority should employ at least twelve home helps for every 1,000 of their local population aged over 65 in order to maintain an effective service. Unfortunately, not all of them do, and many have to operate a rationing system, giving priority to those who are in most need. However, if you feel that you need help, you should still apply.

To apply for a home help, you should contact your local social services office. If you have been ill at home, or in hospital, your doctor may decide you could do with some help in the home and refer your case to the social services department, or a social worker might do this. But if you want to make a direct approach, you or a close friend or relative can either telephone or call in at your local social services office, and explain your problem to the home help organiser. It is the organiser's job to find out exactly what your problems are, how much and what kind of help you need, and then to arrange it for you.

Some local authorities charge for this service, but others provide it free of charge. Yet others may provide it free to people receiving income support, but charge people on a 'means test' of their ability to pay. Each local authority may use a different system, so you might find that while you have to pay for your home help, a friend living in a neighbouring borough gets it free of charge. But charges are kept to a reasonable level.

You might be very lucky and find that you live in a district where the social services are pioneering a scheme for 'intensive home care'. This means that they employ specially trained domestic care assistants who can look after very dependent elderly people in their own homes almost round the clock: waking them up in the morning, getting their breakfast, washing and dressing them, doing the housework and shopping, preparing their meals, doing the laundry, putting them to bed in the evening and even sitting with them at night if necessary. Some may live in for short periods. This sort of service is ideal, but not many local authorities provide it yet. However, as the number of frail elderly people is likely to increase as the years go by, so this intensive home care service should become more widespread.

An added advantage of this system is that the home care assistants are trained to observe their elderly charges, to notice any deterioration in their health or capabilities, and to report this to the home help organiser so that medical or nursing help can be organised, if it is necessary. Many home helps and care assistants strike up close friendships with their 'clients', who get to know and trust them really well. Most home helps are women, but some men take on this work and are very useful in doing redecoration and other odd jobs around the house.

Meals-on-wheels

If getting out to do the shopping and cooking a meal every day are a problem, it is tempting to live on cups of tea and bread and butter or tinned soup and baked beans; but this is not at all good for you. You need a good hot meal of meat or fish and vegetables, plus fruit or a pudding every day, to give you proper nourishment.

By providing a meals-on-wheels service, the social services are making another contribution towards helping you to stay in your own home. The service may be provided in different ways, usually in co-operation with voluntary organisations like the Women's Royal Voluntary Service (WRVS). The meals are generally prepared on local authority premises and delivered by a voluntary worker, but it may be the other way round, or the local authority may make a grant to the voluntary organisation to do the whole job. A charge is made for the meal, which is usually collected by the person delivering the meal. These voluntary workers also get to know their regular customers, and will keep an eye on their general welfare and let the right people know if they need more help. And if you are an elderly person living alone who doesn't have many visitors, it is good to have a regular human contact like this.

To find out more about your local meals-on-wheels service and whether you are eligible for it, contact the local social services office, and talk to the social worker on duty, who will then pass you on to the person responsible. Meals-on-wheels are usually only provided at lunch time, not in the evening, usually only on a weekday, and may only be available on certain days. You may encounter some difficulty if you are a vegetarian or on a special diet, if you belong to an ethnic or religious minority and prefer food you are accustomed to. In the latter case some local authorities make grants to ethnic minority groups, so that they can supply a meal service to the members of their communities.

Lunch clubs, day centres, and day hospitals

A number of local authorities and voluntary organisations run lunch clubs for the elderly, usually on their own premises, where elderly people can come for a good hot meal. They may also provide transport to and from the club for those who can't get about easily, or who can't manage the distance.

Day centres are also provided by local authorities and voluntary groups, usually in separate accommodation but sometimes on the premises of warden-supervised flats or old people's homes. These are places where you can come for the whole day, get coffee, lunch, and tea, and take part in a variety of activities designed to help you occupy your time enjoyably. There may be a keep-fit class, for instance, or an occupational therapy room where you can learn to paint or make toys or rugs, knit or sew, do some indoor gardening or woodwork or take up some other hobby which gives you pleasure and satisfaction. There are likely to be sing-songs, games, bingo sessions, and outings of various kinds. A hairdresser may call regularly, and possibly also a chiropodist. Some private homes and organisations also provide day centres.

Day centres are different from day hospitals, which are usually attached to large hospitals, and run by the health authority. They provide medical and nursing care, as well as physiotherapy, occupational therapy, and speech therapy. Someone who has had a stroke, for example, would probably start attending the day hospital while he was still in hospital, and continue going there after being discharged, so that the treatment could continue for as long as necessary.

Day centres are staffed and run by social services or voluntary organisations employees. Transport is usually provided, either by minibus or by voluntary car drivers, and people are collected from their homes and driven to the centre, and taken home again at the end of the day. A charge is sometimes made for attendance at the centre, usually covering meals and transport, but once again, it is reasonable. To find out more about what is available in your area, contact your local social services office.

Aids and adaptations

If, like Mary Jones, you happen to be crippled with rheumatoid arthritis, there are all sorts of gadgets especially designed to make life easier for you. There are long-lever handles which can be attached to your taps to make them easier to turn; special cutlery which is easy to hold if your fingers are affected; devices to help put on your socks, stockings, and shoes if you find it difficult to bend down; and special fastenings for clothing if you can't do up buttons or zips. These are just a few examples; there are many more.

Your home, too, can be adapted and pieces of equipment installed, such as grab-rails for your stairs, toilet and bathroom; aids to help you get in and out of the bath; or a stair-lift to help you get up and down stairs. If you need to use a wheelchair, doors can be widened so that the chair can get through easily, ramps can be laid over steps so that your chair can run smoothly over them, and rails can be installed round your toilet to enable you to move yourself out of your chair, on to the lavatory, and back again. Age Concern England's booklet *Owning Your Home in Retirement* will give you helpful advice.

A great deal of ingenuity has gone into designing for the disabled, and there is an enormous range of such aids and adaptations. An organisation called the Disabled Living Foundation has a comprehensive exhibition of aids on display at its London premises, where trained staff can take their patients to choose the right aids for them. The acknowledged expert on aids and adaptations is the occupational therapist. Social services departments employ occupational therapists on their staff to visit people in their homes, find out what their problems are, decide what aids and adaptations they need, and arrange for them to be delivered or the work to be carried out. However, you might find that there is a long waiting list in your area, but don't be put off from asking.

Once again, there is great variation between local authorities about the funds they have available for aids and adaptations, and there is often a shortage of occupational therapists, but you should not hesitate to apply to your local social services office if you think something like this would help you. A letter from your GP would give support to your case. You can also buy aids from large chemists. A simple and often cheap piece of equipment, installed with professional advice, can make the world of difference to your daily life and help you to feel in control again.

Other services

These are the main personal social services to which frail old people are entitled, but there are others, such as the laundry service for those whose bedding frequently gets soiled because they are unfortunate enough to be incontinent. Where an old person is being looked after by a relative, there is a scheme called Respite Care, under which the elderly person can be admitted to a residential home for a short period – a couple of weeks, perhaps – to give the caring relative a break and the chance to take a holiday. In some areas, there are schemes for 'fostering' older people with families for short periods, and sometimes on a long-term basis. Hospitals, too, may admit older patients for two weeks at a time to give their caring relative a break.

Some local authorities are now providing telephones and alarm call systems for old people living alone, so that they can call for help in an emergency. There are several different kinds of alarm call system, from the simple to the sophisticated, but they are all connected via telephone or radio to a central switchboard whose operators find out what the problem is, if possible, and then call the right emergency service. These systems are also available privately.

As well as the Respite Care schemes operated by social services departments and hospitals, voluntary organisations such as Age Concern, the Women's Royal Voluntary Service, and the British Red Cross Society provide a 'sitting' service so that carers can take a welcome evening off, and they may also help with shopping and other chores. There are also two organisations whose specific purpose is to give support and advice to carers: one is the Association of Carers and the other the National Council for Carers and Their Elderly Dependants. They work very closely together and help to form local Carers' Support Groups, giving information about what facilities are available locally. It is their intention to merge into one organization in the near future.

Finance

The financial aspects of all this are, of course, vitally important. You should find leaflets in your local post office explaining what financial help you are entitled to, and your local social services office will also send a social worker to discuss your financial affairs in confidence with you, and decide what help you can get. But it is very important to remember that, if you are not satisfied with the charges made for any of these personal social services, you can appeal to the supervisor or person in charge of your social services office, because he has it in his power to negotiate with you, and to overrule decisions made by junior colleagues.

The financial problems people have to cope with in their old age are the subject of a book in themselves, and Age Concern England produces two excellent annual publications full of practical advice and information. They are *Your Rights: A Guide to Benefits for Retired People*, and *Your Taxes and Savings in Retirement*.

Health services

Your GP is the chief person responsible for looking after your health and for arranging nursing care and treatment in your home if you need it. For example, if you need nursing care, he will contact the district nursing service or arrange for you to be visited by district nurses attached to his practice. Some group practices have health visitors attached to them. Health visitors work mainly with children, but some are now specialising in working with elderly people, which is a good move. They may visit them in their homes regularly – not just when they are ill – to check on their health and welfare, and with their trained eyes will spot a problem at its earliest stage and prevent it from getting out of hand by reporting it to the doctor and arranging what treatment may be necessary. Unfortunately not nearly enough health visitors are yet doing this specialised work.

The district nursing service is also hard-pressed, and district nurses are not always able to give the sort of service they would like. But they are dedicated people who take a great interest in their older patients; many of them take special training courses in nursing the elderly, as this age group forms a large part of their case-load.

For those who are able to pay for private nursing, there are many nursing agencies which supply trained nurses for short or long periods to nurse people in their own homes; and there are two charitable organisations which supply specialised nursing care to supplement the district nursing service, for those who are terminally ill and want to die at home. These organisations are the Marie Curie Memorial Foundation, and the Macmillan Nursing Service, both of which provide at reasonable cost nurses with special training in care of the dying. As you can imagine, this is very demanding work, but these nurses are wonderfully committed to helping their patients to a peaceful and pain-free death, and to supporting the bereaved relatives.

If you have any problems with your doctor – and there are good and bad doctors just as there are good and bad builders or plumbers – you should contact your local Family Practitioner Committee. It is known, for instance, that some GPs are reluctant to take elderly patients on to their lists, or to visit them at home. If this should happen to you, and you want to complain about it or to find another, more helpful, doctor, you should get in touch with your Family Practitioner Committee, whose address will be in the local telephone directory, and explain your problem to them.

If you don't get any satisfaction from your Family Practitioner Committee, you can take your complaint to your Community Health Council, an independent body representing the public which can take issues up with the local health authority. If you don't get satisfaction from your health authority, you can, as a last resort, take your case to the Health Service Ombudsman, who, if he thinks your complaint is valid, will investigate it and report his findings. He will also request that action be taken to put things right, if he considers you have been wrongly treated. His powers only extend to administrative matters, however, not to matters of clinical judgment. These are dealt with by the General Medical Council, or – in the case of nurses – by the UK Central Council for Nursing, Midwifery, and Health Visiting. The addresses are listed at the back of this book.

A good family doctor, however, will give you not only all the medical care you need, but also information about other services you may find helpful, such as a local club for victims of stroke, Age Concern, or a local branch of Cruse, for example. There are usually notices about clubs and societies which offer help of all kinds in doctors' waiting rooms and surgeries, and they are well worth following up. A number of charitable organisations, such as Age Concern, the Women's Royal Voluntary Service (WRVS), and the British Red Cross Society (BRCS), provide all kinds of services and facilities to elderly disabled people. Their head office address is listed at the back of this publication, and Age Concern, the WRVS, and the BRCS have local groups which will be listed in the telephone directory. It is well worth contacting them if you have a particular problem, because they might be able to help, or perhaps pass you on to someone who can. If English is not your first language, and you are not very fluent, you should try to get an interpreter, possibly from social services. If you are in London you may get one from the Standing Conference of Ethnic Minority Senior Citizens (address at back of this book).

James Green was a widower of 72, who lived alone in a council flat. One day he had a stroke, which left him with one arm paralysed and some difficulty with speech. He was given physiotherapy, occupational therapy, and speech therapy while he was in hospital, all of which helped him a great deal, but he was not sure how he would manage when he got home. The hospital occupational therapist and physiotherapist took him on a visit to his flat to see what gadgets and other adaptations he would need, and arranged for them to be installed before he was discharged. A member of the British Red Cross Society visited him in hospital, asked if there was anyone to look after him at home, and when she found there wasn't, she arranged for someone to clean, air, and warm up his flat and see that there was enough food in his larder. When he got home, he found that he could manage quite well with the special gadgets he had been given. He was also put in touch with a local 'Stroke Club', run by the Chest, Heart, and Stroke Association, which he could attend once a week and meet other people like himself who had suffered strokes, and be given help with any difficulties he might have from time to time. The local authority had installed an alarm call system in his flat, so he felt safe in the knowledge that he could call for help in an emergency.

A home help called three days a week to do the chores for him, and he was able to go to the local day centre for a meal and some company during the week. He was lucky in having good neighbours, who kept an eye on him at weekends, and he managed to stay in his own home in spite of his disabilities. He was full of spirit and determination, as well as humour, which all helped to see him through his difficulties.

Chapter three

Are there any alternatives to going into a home?

If you are still reasonably active, but find that going on living in your present home is, for one reason or another, just not possible, there are two main alternatives to consider before thinking about moving into a 'home'. One alternative is to go and live with your family and the other to move into sheltered accommodation.

Moving in with the family

If you have children who are married and living in a large house, the most obvious solution to your problem would seem to be to move in with them, so that they can keep an eye on you, and look after you when you need it. You would be part of a family again, there might be youngsters around for you to enjoy, you would be able to make your own contribution to family life, and you would feel secure in knowing there was someone to rely on in your old age.

But this sort of arrangement needs a lot of careful thought and discussion beforehand if it is to work well. Both you and your son or daughter must be absolutely frank with each other, and you must also bring your son's wife or daughter's husband into the discussion as part of your family. Nor must you forget to be absolutely honest with yourself, when you are considering all the aspects and the possible difficulties, before you take this step. Relationships can only too easily turn sour if all the practicalities have not been thoroughly thrashed out and mutually agreed, and if there is not enough trust and 'give and take' on both sides.

Not so long ago it was accepted that all the generations would live together in what is known as the 'extended family', with the grandparents (or oldest generation) being accorded the honoured position of head of the family. This is still the case in some parts of the world. Nowadays – in Western society at least – the family has split up into small units, and it is rare to find them all living together under one roof.

In going to live with the family, older people cannot expect to be given a position of priority as a matter of course; if you accept this, it will be easier to work out together what your relationship will be. Both you and your children will be used to having your own independence, and neither of you will want to surrender it completely. The first thing to do, then, will be to agree on the degree of independence each of you can and should retain, to allow you to lead separate lives when you want to without creating practical problems or offending each other in any way. You will also need to discuss, with tact and sensitivity on both sides, how far you can get involved in family life; there is nothing worse than a grandparent who keeps interfering with the upbringing of young children, or the running of the house.

Some families solve the relationship problem by building on, or converting part of the house to, a 'granny flat' or annexe. This may be an excellent solution in some cases, as it provides both closeness and access to the family when needed, and at the same time independence in one's own surroundings. Having one's own front door is a great boon at times! But it is wise to have a legal agreement drawn up between you about ownership or tenancy of the accommodation, as there is always the possibility that the couple whose house you are living in may split up, or divorce, or that the husband gets a new job in a different part of the country, or even that they may want to emigrate and start life anew elsewhere. Then the house would have to be sold, you would have to find somewhere else to live, and you might have a financial problem on your hands.

If the house is not large enough for a flat or annexe, the answer may be to have your own bed-sittingroom, with washing and cooking facilities, so that you can entertain your own visitors, or keep yourself to yourself and not intrude on your family, whose privacy you must also respect. It is vital to have a carefully thought-out agreement about the degree to which family life can be shared, and stick to it. The older generation have to learn to be tolerant of the young, and the young to understand the problems and difficulties of the old.

It is worth remembering that there is often a very real affinity between the very old and the very young; grandparents often develop a special relationship with their grandchildren and become great companions with them. At the same time, one hears all too many stories of older people going to live with younger relatives and being made to feel lonely and unwanted, and excluded from family life.

> ***Fred James*** was a bachelor, in his early eighties, who after he retired from teaching lived with his two unmarried sisters in the family house in Scotland. His sisters were both older than he was, and after they died he was left alone in a house which was much too big for him. He had also had a recent colostomy, which at times he found difficult to manage.
>
> Fred had two nieces, one married with a large family, the other single, who both asked him to go and live with them. The single niece lived on her own in London, while the married niece lived with her husband and two children in a large family house in a northern university town. Now that the older children had grown up and left home, the house was being converted into bed-sittingrooms which could be let to students during term time. Fred decided to live with his married niece, as a tenant in one of the bed-sittingrooms.

He thought he would be lonely in London, far away from his native land, particularly as his niece had to work and he would be alone all day; whereas with his married niece he would be part of a large family, able to enjoy their comings and goings and the company of different generations. He would also be able to retreat to the privacy of his own room when he wanted to.

Fred settled into his new life very well, and soon became a valued member of the family. After a lifetime as a teacher he was very good at handling young people, and the younger members of the family often turned to him for help and advice. When he fell ill his niece nursed him devotedly. There was give and take on both sides: he was able to enjoy a happy family life and care when he needed it, while his financial contribution and his help with the domestic and gardening chores was much appreciated. Fred had made the right choice.

Sheltered accommodation

If you have no younger relatives, or if you prefer to remain independent of them, you might consider moving to what is called 'sheltered' housing or accommodation. This is housing – usually self-contained flats or bungalows – which is specially designed for older people who want to live independently in a home of their own but who need the security of someone at hand in emergencies, and communal facilities to make life easier and more enjoyable. This sort of housing is usually in a large purpose-built complex with communal gardens, lounges, laundry facilities, and usually with one or more guest rooms where visitors can stay overnight, and sometimes a dining-room and kitchen. There should be a warden on hand throughout the day and night, living on the premises, to keep an eye on residents, be available to them in emergencies, and generally be concerned with their welfare.

Each unit of this type of accommodation should be equipped with an adequate alarm call system so that the residents can call the warden in an emergency, such as a fall or a fainting fit. There should be hand-rails on all the stairs and in corridors, grabrails in toilets and bathrooms, electric points at waist height so that they can be reached without bending down, long handles on doors and taps which are easy to turn, doors wide enough to allow a wheelchair or walking-frame through, and cookers, sinks, and working surfaces all at an easy height for working.

There is some local authority housing of this kind, about which your local housing department can give you details, although waiting lists are normally long, and every council has its own allocations policy, taking into account people's physical and social needs. In addition to this, a number of housing associations have rented accommodation including sheltered housing. A growing number of private companies are also building sheltered housing for sale in some areas.

There is a lot to be said for this type of accommodation. It will give you independence, security, convenient facilities, and the companionship of other residents when you want it. But there are several points to be considered.

First, it is important to try and find such accommodation in your own area, or one that you know well, so that you are among friends and in familiar surroundings.

Second, it should be conveniently situated, near the town centre so that you can easily reach the post office and other shops, library, bus routes, railway station, your doctor's surgery, parks, gardens, and places of entertainment. Too many sheltered housing complexes are built in isolated areas on the outskirts of a town, so that residents are remote from the rest of the community and find it difficult to establish social contacts. There is a danger that 'ghettos' are being created where elderly residents are to all intents and purposes immured together, without much contact with the outside world.

Third, you should make sure that a sheltered flat or bungalow you are considering is properly equipped for an older person – not only for your present needs, but for any you may have in the future. Some social services departments are being inundated with requests for aids and adaptations in privately built sheltered housing which should have been included in the original design.

Fourth, you have to remember that though the warden is there to help residents in every way he or she can, and particularly in emergencies, she cannot take care of you when you are ill. You will need the same medical and nursing care that you would in your own home, and if you fall seriously ill, or become very disabled, you may have to face another move – into hospital, or a nursing home or rest home.

Fifth, you may have a much-loved pet, and find that pets are not permitted in your sheltered flat, so that you have to face parting with it.

Sixth, sheltered housing is not cheap to buy, and you have to bear in mind that there will also be a service charge to pay to cover the warden's salary; the upkeep of the premises; heat, light, and power for the communal areas; water rates; and any other services that may be provided. Service charges average between £8 and £15 a week at 1988 prices.

Extra-care sheltered housing

Some councils and housing associations (but only one or two private companies) have a form of sheltered housing with additional services such as meals and higher staffing levels. These schemes are intended to help residents to remain as independent as possible by providing additional help with personal care. Nursing is not usually provided.

This housing is sometimes called 'very sheltered housing' or 'extra-care sheltered housing' and is for people who find that although they need more support than sheltered housing usually offers, they do not need to go into a residential home.

For more information about sheltered accommodation, you should write to Age Concern England, which produces fact sheets on the subject (send a large SAE and state whether you are interested in renting or buying), and also publishes a very useful booklet called *Buyer's Guide to Sheltered Housing*.

Geraldine Jameson lived with her husband in a large house just outside Manchester. When he died she found the house much too large for her to manage on her own, and as she suffered badly from asthma she decided to move to a warden-supervised flat in a seaside town on the south coast which was said to be ideal for asthmatics. When she moved in, she found that most of her furniture was much too large for the rather small rooms, so she had to get rid of it and buy new furniture. Although her flat was comfortable, and there was every amenity she needed, she found it cramped and dark after her lovely big house, and also it was situated away from the town centre, so that she had to hire a taxi whenever she went into town, as she got breathless if she walked far. This was not only expensive, but it also meant she could not get out as much as she liked, or join societies and participate in their activities. After only a few months Mrs Jameson found that she bitterly regretted moving away from her home, and her asthma got worse, not better, because she was worried and unhappy. Eventually she decided to cut her losses and go back to Manchester, where she fortunately found a sheltered housing scheme very near the area where she used to live, so she was back among her friends again and settled down happily.

Chapter four

Are there different kinds of home to choose from?

Having thought carefully about these three possibilities – staying at home with extra help, moving in with your family, or moving into sheltered housing – you may still feel for one reason or another that going into a home is for you the best solution. If so, you will want to know more about what kinds of home are available, and what they have to offer, before you make your final decision. The rest of this book will tell you as much as possible about the different types of home there are, who runs them, what laws exist to ensure they don't fall below an acceptable standard, how much they cost and how you can pay, what protections residents have against abuse of any kind, and how to set about finding one that is suited to your needs and will offer you a good quality of life. This chapter concentrates on the different types of homes there are to choose from.

To begin with, homes can be divided into two main categories: residential care homes, and nursing homes. Residential care homes are also known as 'old people's homes', 'rest homes', or 'eventide homes' if they cater specifically for elderly people. They may, of course, cater for other groups of people such as those who are mentally handicapped, or who are addicted to drugs or alcohol and who need special care, but a large proportion of them specialise in caring for the elderly.

Residential care homes provide care of the kind that a relative would give: that is to say, help with getting up in the morning, washing, dressing, going to the toilet, having a bath, and so on. They are suitable for people who can't manage on their own at home, but who don't require skilled nursing. Someone who does need constant attention by trained nurses will have to go into a nursing home, which by law has to be managed by a qualified doctor or nurse, and staffed by qualified nurses.

There are a few homes which provide both types of care. Usually the main residential care home has rooms where residents can be nursed by trained nurses if they fall ill. Some homes may have a nursing unit or wing, but this means that the resident has to move out of his or her room and – if the home is a private one – may have to pay extra to keep it unoccupied by another resident. It is obviously ideal if the resident can be nursed in his own room, without having to move out of familiar surroundings. Such homes are still very few and far between, however, and it is to be hoped their number will increase.

Both residential care and nursing homes must, under the law, be registered, but they come under different authorities. Residential care homes are the responsibility of the local authority, while nursing homes come under the health authority. What registration means, and why it is necessary, is explained in the next chapter. For the moment, let's look at these two types of home in more detail.

Residential care homes

It is a far cry from the old days when the needy could expect to end their days in that forbidding institution, the workhouse. Nowadays there is an enormously wide range of accommodation for elderly people in need of care: some homes are provided and run by local authorities, some by charitable organisations, and an increasing number by private companies and individuals. We shall consider each group separately.

Local authority homes

Old people's homes provided by local authorities are intended for those living in the locality who cannot continue living at home because they are frail or disabled, and who are on low incomes. It was the National Assistance Act (1948) which first laid down that local authorities must provide residential accommodation 'for persons who by reason of age, infirmity, and any other circumstances are in need of care and attention which is not otherwise available to them'. This clause is included in Part III of the Act, which is why such homes are often referred to as 'Part III accommodation'. (These homes are known as Part IV in Scotland after the relevant section of the Social Work (Scotland) Act 1968.)

Local authority homes vary enormously in size and quality, just as other homes do. They may be modern and purpose-built, or they may be converted older houses; they are usually fairly large, taking between 20 and 50 residents. There should be some single and double rooms, where residents can take their own possessions, but in some local authority homes there are still rooms for three or four people.

The staff running these homes are employed by the social services department of the local authority. The Head of the Home is usually a senior social worker, with a deputy and a staff of care assistants to look after the residents, as well as the usual domestic workers. Staff should encourage the residents to be active and independent, to have visitors and to go on outings, and to enjoy their own hobbies and leisure interests. Some homes have a bar where residents can buy and enjoy a drink when they feel like it, and a small shop where they can purchase necessities if they can't get out to the local shops.

If you want to apply for a place in a local authority residential home, you should contact your local social services office, where the social worker on duty will refer your request to the person responsible for handling such applications. A social worker will then come to see you and discuss your problems with you, find out what your circumstances are, and exactly what sort of help you need. After considering this information, the social services department will decide whether or not they can offer you a place in a home. If they do, your name will be added to the waiting list – there is nearly always a waiting list for places – and it may be many months before there is a vacancy.

Places are normally allotted only to people who have lived in the local authority area for a specified period of time, and although some local authorities do accept applications from other areas, you are likely to find it very difficult to get a place in a local authority home outside your own district, if you want to be near your family, for example. In any case, you will normally need the support of the local authority in whose area you live. Because waiting lists are long, it is unlikely that you will have a choice of which home to go into; you have to take what is offered. You should, however, expect to be able to see the home and spend some time there before you make your decision. In most cases the first month is regarded as a trial period from both sides. If you are really unhappy in the home to which you have been allocated, you can ask to be transferred to another home, but this too is bound to take time.

Each local authority fixes a standard weekly charge for the homes in its own area, based on the actual running costs. If you can't afford to pay this charge, the social services department will assess how much you can afford to pay, and charge you this sum. Chapter 9 goes into all the details of charges for residential care, and how these can be met.

Jim Smith had worked on the railways all his life, but had to retire when a circulatory disorder got so bad he had to have a leg amputated. He never managed to walk very well with his artificial leg, but his wife looked after him and made life easy. Then she died suddenly from a heart attack, and Jim found himself unable to cope on his own at home. His GP, who kept an eye on him, contacted the social services and asked them to admit him to a residential home. A social worker called to see him, found he had only his state pension and occupational pension to live on, with hardly any savings to fall back on. He rented his house from the council. The social services department found him a place in a home quite near his house, so that he could keep in touch with his friends and neighbours, and charged him just as much as he could afford to pay. They thought it wise to admit him as soon as possible, as his good leg was showing signs of trouble and making it even more difficult for him to get about. He found it difficult to adjust to his new life at first, but settled down when he began to make new friends in the home.

Voluntary homes

A number of voluntary organisations and charitable bodies provide homes for the elderly on a non-profit-making basis. The charges vary according to the facilities the home offers, but are usually reasonable, being based on running costs, with any profits being ploughed back into improving the quality of the accommodation and the care and facilities provided. Such homes may be run by charities, religious organisations, or by professional associations for their retired members.

To get a place in a voluntary home you have to prove that you meet the conditions that the particular organisation lays down. You may also have to give details of your financial situation, and possibly also have a medical examination.

Voluntary homes vary considerably in size; some are small with fewer than ten residents, while others are large enough to take 100 people. Rooms may be single or shared. Priority for places is according to need – both financial and physical – with the result that waiting lists can be long.

Some charitable organisations provide a full range of sheltered accommodation for the elderly: warden-supervised housing, rest homes, and nursing facilities. An example is Nightingale House, in Clapham, south London, which is the largest home for Jewish old people in Europe. It can accommodate an old person in the type of housing and with the degree of care suited to his needs right up to the end of his life. An individual or a married couple can apply first for a warden-supervised flat and when they can no longer look after themselves they may be moved into the rest home building, where there are communal dining rooms, lounges, a library, recreational therapy, gardens, a small synagogue, and medical facilities, with a medical supervisor, full-time matron, and visiting doctors, dentist, chiropodist, eye specialist, physiotherapist, and occupational therapist. There is a nursing wing where anyone who falls ill can be cared for by trained nurses.

This type of comprehensive complex is similar to that pioneered in Denmark in the 1960s, and provided by the State for all elderly people in need of care and support. There are advantages and disadvantages, of course. The main advantage is that a resident does not have to face the trauma of moving out of his familiar surroundings when he becomes too dependent on others to stay where he is, but can stay in the place and among people he knows, right up to the end of his life. The main disadvantage is that such large complexes of accommodation for the old and frail can become isolated from the local community, so that the residents are segregated from the rest of society.

Some charitable bodies and professional associations are building residential homes with nursing units attached, so that they can provide what is being called 'total care'. Others, such as the Abbeyfield Society, are providing 'extra care' homes, where the care assistants are trained to give that little bit extra attention to heavily disabled residents as described in the previous chapter.

Joan Robinson had worked in the Civil Service all her life, employed by the DHSS. She had lived with her mother for many years in the family house, and moved into a small flat after her mother died. She was single, but was very active, with many friends, and took it badly when she developed arthritis in her hips and had to have one replaced. As she got older she became less and less mobile and able to look after herself, and began to think the time had come to go into a home. She had belonged to the Civil Service Association all her working life and knew they had some very nice rest homes in different parts of the country, so wrote a letter of application for a place in one of them. After some weeks she was offered a choice of two homes – a new one which had just been built in Scotland, and a converted old mansion in Sussex. Having spent much of her life in London she chose Sussex, both because it was nearer and because it had a small nursing wing, and was set in beautiful grounds. She was given a room of her own where she could take her own furniture and possessions, and with a tiny bathroom adjoining it. She settled comfortably and decided she had been very lucky. The room was not cheap, but with a good pension and some money in the bank she could afford to pay for it without keeping herself short of cash.

Private homes

There has been a tremendous boom in the supply of privately owned rest homes over the past few years as both individuals and companies, with capital to invest, saw the potential profits to be made from providing accommodation and care for the ever-increasing elderly population. Some of these private owners were honest and reputable, offering homes with a high degree of comfort and care. Others were less reputable, concerned only with making a profit and unscrupulous about how they exploited their vulnerable elderly residents in order to do so. Scandals were reported in the Press and stories related of overcrowding, dirt, lack of facilities, residents' pension books being appropriated, confused elderly people being locked in their rooms and even restrained in their beds or chairs, and general ill treatment and threats for anyone who complained.

At this time the law was so lax that anyone with a house offering accommodation for four or more people could apply to the local authority to become a registered home-owner, and there were few – if any – safeguards to ensure that rest home proprietors and managers were suitable people for this responsibility. Registration fees were, at £1, so laughably low that local authorities could not afford to finance and administer regular inspection of these homes, with the result that the standards of some of them were abysmal.

The Government reacted to the situation by overhauling the legislation governing standards in both residential care and nursing homes, bringing the two together under one legal umbrella in the form of the Registered Homes Act 1984, which came into force in January 1985. Under this Act more stringent conditions for registration were introduced, and registration fees were increased to a level which was intended to cover the costs of administration and inspection. A Code of Practice was also produced on behalf of the Government by the Centre for Policy on Ageing, for use by both registering authorities and home owners and managers, to give guidelines on the rights residents are entitled to expect and the care they should expect to receive. The new legislation is explained fully in the next chapter.

It should not be difficult to find a private rest home if you live in a 'retirement' area, but it might be more of a problem if you live in the heart of the country or in an inner city area. A greater problem will lie in choosing the right one. The standards of some homes have always been high; others have raised their standards in accordance with the new Act; but there are inevitably still a few which leave a lot to be desired. Later chapters in this book offer advice on how to start looking for a home, what to look for when you are visiting possible homes, and what your rights are under the Code of Practice.

Charges for rooms in private homes vary enormously, from about £90 a week up to £300 and over. But a high price does not necessarily indicate high quality – you can be miserable in luxury and happy in modest surroundings. What really matters is the attitude of the home's manager and staff.

Michael Gray and his wife Sue had his his mother living with them until she began to get confused and difficult in her behaviour, as well as incontinent. They looked for a residential home which would take her and where she would be properly looked after. Eventually they found one which seemed suitable as it was managed by a woman who said she was a qualified nurse who specialised in looking after confused elderly people. It was a pleasant house with nice gardens, and large rooms – but there were five or six residents in each room, and very little privacy. The manager said this was necessary, as it was wrong to leave this type of resident on their own: they needed company and constant supervision. She also asked them not to come and visit her too soon, to give her time to settle down, so they left it for a month before coming to see her. They were shocked to find her much worse than she had been, her clothes and bedding stained with urine, her hair uncombed, and looking thin and undernourished. She had obviously been completely neglected. After a fierce argument with the manager, they took her back home with them, and sent for the family doctor. He immediately arranged for her to go into hospital while they looked around for a much better home for her. They also reported the home to the local authority, and asked them to investigate it.

Nursing homes

The term 'nursing home' covers a wide variety of establishments, from large private hospitals and clinics to small homes for half-a-dozen patients, many of which specialise in health care of the elderly. In recent years the number of elderly patients needing long-term care has increased and some health authorities have made contract arrangements with nursing homes to take hospital patients who still require nursing care but no longer need all the facilities available in a hospital. In these circumstances the health authority remains responsible for the payment of fees and agrees the rates with the nursing home owners. However, only a few health authorities have this type of contractual arrangement.

National Health Service homes

The NHS is also experimenting with providing its own nursing homes for 'long-stay patients' – elderly people who require long-term nursing care. Three experimental NHS homes have been set up – one outside Sheffield, one near Portsmouth, and the third at Fleetwood in Lancashire. In these homes most patients have their own rooms, though there are double rooms for those who want to share. The Head of Home is a senior nurse, who is in full charge of the running of the home, with a staff of trained nurses and nursing auxiliaries, domestics and voluntary workers. Medical care is provided by local GPs, who visit regularly. The communal rooms – the dining-room and the lounge – are pleasant; social events and visitors are encouraged, and patients who are sufficiently fit and mobile are taken on shopping expeditions and outings to places of interest. Residents are also encouraged to participate in running the home through a residents' committee. The aim is to make these nursing homes very much part of their local communities, and as much of a 'home from home' as possible.

These experimental homes are being evaluated over a period of five years, after which presumably a decision will be taken as to whether or not other similar homes should be set up, perhaps on a nationwide basis. It is significant, perhaps, that already a number of health authorities are establishing their own nursing homes for the elderly, without waiting for the results of this experiment to be evaluated and made known. They are already convinced of their value. However, for the time being, the chances of finding one in your area are slender.

Voluntary nursing homes

The situation regarding nursing homes owned by voluntary organisations is much as it is for rest homes. But there are not many of them, and they tend to reserve their beds for residents from their own rest homes who need nursing care. Waiting lists are, therefore, usually very long.

Voluntary nursing homes have to be registered with the district health authority, as do privately owned nursing homes. Fees are reasonable, as charitable organisations are non-profit-making, but anyone who cannot afford them can apply for financial help to the local social security office.

Private nursing homes

There has been a boom in the number of privately owned nursing homes, too, and many of them are catering specifically for older patients. Private nursing homes have been under much stricter regulations than private residential homes, with the result that general standards are considerably higher. Again, the sizes of homes and fees charged for rooms and nursing care vary enormously.

The law lays down that private nursing homes must be managed by a qualified doctor or nurse, and that they must be registered with the district health authority, or health board in Scotland, which must inspect them regularly to monitor their standards. Since 1981, registration fees have been much higher than those for rest homes, and inspection procedures more regular and stringent. The Registered Homes Act 1984 has in fact brought residential care homes into line with nursing homes from this point of view.

Peter Freeman had two serious strokes in quick succession, which left him paralysed on one side of his body, incontinent, and with a severe speech defect. Aged 76, he was a large, heavy man, and his wife, who was only a year younger and suffered from arthritis, knew she wouldn't be able to nurse him at home. When the time came near for him to be discharged from hospital, the consultant geriatrician in charge of the ward discussed Peter's future with her frankly and sympathetically. He couldn't be expected to get much better, he said, and while he wasn't acutely ill now, he would need good nursing care for the rest of his life. He suggested finding a room for Peter in a private nursing home. The hospital social worker helped them to find a nursing home quite near Peter and Amy's house, so she could visit him frequently without too much difficulty. As Peter was entitled to supplementary benefit, the nursing home could recover the weekly fees from the DHSS, on their scale of charges. Peter would be able to pay for any extra facilities he needed out of his own pocket. Amy went to see the home before they made their decision, and liked it. The Matron seemed a very pleasant and capable person, and the atmosphere in the home was cheerful and friendly. Peter was discharged from hospital into the nursing home, where he was well looked after by the staff of trained nurses and auxiliaries. Amy was very relieved, as she had been extremely worried about the future.

Homes for religious and ethnic minorities

People who belong to the Jewish community are well catered for through the activities of the Jewish Welfare Board (see the address at the back of this book). In Leeds, for example, there are four sheltered housing schemes, as well as flats for elderly tenants on an estate developed by the Leeds Jewish Housing Association. The London Jewish Welfare Board runs fourteen homes, some linked with sheltered housing, and there is Nightingale House in Clapham, the largest Jewish Old People's Home in Europe, with nearly 400 places, which comprises sheltered flats, a large residential home with all sorts of amenities, including a small synagogue, and a nursing home. Here residents can move from one type of accommodation to another according to their needs, yet remain in their familiar surroundings and among their friends.

Other ethnic and religious groups are not yet so well served, although the Asian, Afro-Caribbean, and Cypriot communities have initiated various schemes for housing their frail old people. Much remains to be done, however, and in particular the local authorities need to become much more aware of the special needs of different minority groups, in the way of diet, language, and customs. It must be rare, for example, for the meals-on-wheels service to provide food acceptable to a Hindu or Moslem whose religion forbids him to eat certain things.

Indira Patel had come to England from East Africa with her husband and two children about twenty years ago. They had settled in the East Midlands, where there was quite a large Asian community, and Mr Patel had had no difficulty in finding a job and earning enough to keep them all. They were also lucky enough to find a council flat, and Indira stayed at home to run the house and look after her family while her husband went out to work and her children to school. As they were living among other Asians, she only learned to speak enough English to find her way by bus to the town centre and to do her shopping. Her husband looked after all their business and personal affairs, so Indira had no need to learn to read or write English.

After they had grown up and left school, the two children decided to go to Canada, where friends of theirs had found jobs, so Indira and her husband were left on their own. It was a terrible shock to Indira when her husband had a sudden heart attack and died within a few days, leaving her alone. She coped somehow, with the help of friends and neighbours, until one day she had a bad fall while out shopping, broke her leg in several places, and was told by the hospital doctors she would have difficulty in walking again, at her age, and should think about going into a home.

Being used to letting others take the initiative, Indira allowed the hospital social worker to find her a place in a local authority home, and obediently moved in there, but found she was the only Asian resident. No one spoke her language or understood her customs, the food was all English – which she disliked; and she found it difficult to communicate with both the staff and other residents. As a result she was extremely lonely and unhappy, and felt totally out of place. When a former neighbour called in to see her, she poured out her troubles to her. The next day her neighbour's husband came to see her and to tell her about an organisation called ASRA (Asian Sheltered Residential Accommodation) which was converting old houses in an area nearby into self-contained units for Asian old people, with a resident warden to look after them.

It sounded too good to be true when her neighbour returned a week later to say her husband had put Indira's name on the waiting list for one of these units, so that as soon as one fell vacant she would have the opportunity to take it. In just three months she was able to move into her own small flat, on the ground floor, equipped with all the aids and adaptations which would enable her to cope on her own, but with the warden always on call should she need help. Best of all, she was back among her own people again, able to speak her own language and make new friends.

Chapter five

How does the law protect the public?

The disastrous experience that the Grays had in their attempt to find a 'home from home' for Michael's mother (see page 51) is less likely to happen now that new laws have been passed to protect the public from unscrupulous or incompetent home owners and managers. When the local authority investigated their complaint, they found that the manager was not, in fact, a qualified nurse; neither she nor any of her staff had experience or training in caring for confused elderly people; the standards of hygiene in the home were lamentably low; and there was serious overcrowding and lack of privacy for residents. The home had not been inspected for several years – probably not since it was first registered – so no check had been made on its standards of care. The local authority decided to withdraw its registration certificate, so the home was closed.

It was precisely to prevent this sort of thing from happening that the Registered Homes Act 1984 was introduced. Under this Act, for example, anyone wanting to open a residential or nursing home for the elderly has to prove he is a fit person to do so and any qualifications he claims have to be verified. Someone who opened a home without applying for registration would be committing an offence. FOR THIS REASON THE FIRST THING TO DO WHEN YOU ARE LOOKING FOR A POSSIBLE HOME IS TO MAKE SURE ANY YOU ARE CONSIDERING ARE REGISTERED: A REGISTRATION CERTIFICATE MUST BE DISPLAYED IN A PROMINENT POSITION WHERE IT CAN EASILY BE SEEN BY VISITORS.

A home that is residential in the main but also provides skilled nursing must be registered with both the local authority and the health authority. This is known as 'dual registration'.

What does registration mean?

The registering authority – either the local authority or the district health authority – is responsible for making sure that the standards of residential care and nursing homes are high, and that these homes are properly managed. The registering authority should, therefore, consider each application for registration very carefully before granting it, in order to satisfy themselves that the legal requirements have been fulfilled: that is, that the owner/manager is a fit person to run such a home, that the accommodation is adequate for the proposed number of residents, and that there will be a sufficient number of trained and untrained staff to look after them.

Once a licence has been granted, and the home has been registered, the registering authority must inspect it at regular intervals to see that standards are being kept up and are not allowed to fall to an unacceptable level. If faults are found, the inspector should point them out and ask that they are put right within a specified time. If this is not done to his or her satisfaction, the case should be reported to senior officers of the authority who should then put pressure on the owner and manager to put things right. If these senior officers are still not satisfied that the home is up to standard, they will recommend to the authority that registration be cancelled.

Residential care homes are registered and inspected by officers of the local authority social services department at least once a year and may be increased to twice, and nursing homes by community medical and nursing officers from the district health authority at least twice a year. If a home has dual registration, it must be inspected by a joint team.

Owner/managers are, of course, entitled to appeal against a decision of the registering authority if they consider it unfair. The case will be heard by an independent tribunal of experts including lawyers, doctors, nurses, and social workers, who hear evidence from both sides and may also visit the home and interview the residents and staff to help them arrive at a fair decision. The welfare of residents is, of course, their primary concern.

What does the Act say?

Put briefly, and in simple language, this is what the Act says:

- It is an offence to carry on a home for four or more residents without being registered under the Act. Homes with fewer than four residents need not be registered.

- The registering authority will decide how many residents, and of what sex, the home may accommodate; and it may lay down other conditions of registration as well. The owner/manager is committing an offence if he or she does not comply with these conditions.

- When a home is accepted for registration, the owner/manager must pay an initial fee. A certificate of registration will be issued by the authority, which must be displayed in a conspicuous position in the home (usually in the entrance hall). The owner/manager will also have to pay an annual fee to the registering authority, based on the number of places available in the home.

- The authority can refuse to register a home if the owner/manager or anyone else involved in running the home is considered not to be a fit person; or if the premises or staff are not considered suitable; or if the home will not provide reasonable services or facilities.

- A registration can be cancelled if the owner/manager or

REGISTERED HOMES ACT 1984

Certificate of Registration

East Sussex

Registration No.   Certificate No. 0966

THIS IS TO CERTIFY that

of

has been registered to carry on the business of a home for

at

under the management of

by East Sussex County Council in pursuance of the Registered Homes Act 1984
IT IS A CONDITION of the said registration that*

DATED this   day of   19

Signed: _____

SPECIMEN

TO COUNTY TREASURER'S INCOME SECTION: PERIODICAL INCOME REGISTER
Please add the above named proprietor or organisation to the Periodical Income Register.

An annual fee based on the above number of beds (refer to Social Services Department for the current charge per bed) is payable on the Registration Date shown and on subsequent anniversaries of that date, in advance. An invoice for the first annual fee should be issued as soon as possible.

The Registration Number above should form the last 3 digits of the PIR reference and will be quoted by the inspectorate in future correspondence.

*Insert, where appropriate, conditions regulating the age, sex or other category of persons who may be received in the home.

SS/358C   CC 978

REGISTRATION FORMS 57

REGISTERED HOMES ACT 1984

Certificate of Registration

THIS IS TO CERTIFY that

of

carrying on a Nursing Home at

has been registered in respect of such home by

under the provisions of the Registered Homes Act 1984

CONDITIONS OF REGISTRATION:

1   The number of persons for whom accommodation is provided at any one time shall not exceed
*

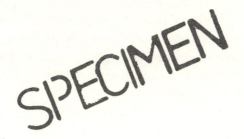

(*Insert any other condition(s) imposed under s. 29 of the Act.)

Signed _____
on behalf of the registration authority
Dated _____ 19 _____   No. _____

THIS CERTIFICATE MUST BE DISPLAYED CONSPICUOUSLY IN THE HOME - FAILURE TO DO SO IS AN OFFENCE.

Cat No. NH 64   © SHAW & SONS LTD., Shaway House, London, SE26 5AE   WQX 00234-1 anyone else involved in running the home has committed any offence under the Act, or has refused to comply with conditions laid down by the registering authority. If there is a serious risk to the life, health, or well-being of residents, the registering authority can apply to a Justice of the Peace for an order to cancel registration immediately.

— The registering authority has to give its reasons for cancelling registration to the owner/manager, who has the right to make representations to the authority and to put his or her case. If the authority sticks to its guns, the owner/manager can appeal to the Registered Homes Tribunal, which will make a final judgment on the matter.

The Act authorises the Secretary of State for Social Services to lay down regulations for running residential care homes, and also authorises the registering authority to inspect the premises at regular intervals. Homes must be inspected at least once a year (this may be changed to twice in 1988), but some authorities inspect them every six months, and some every three months. Anyone who obstructs an inspector in the course of his or her duty is guilty of an offence.

These conditions apply to both residential care and nursing homes, except that the Act specifies that any nursing home, irrespective of size, must be registered; and that it must be managed by a qualified doctor or nurse.

What all this means is that residents in registered residential care and nursing homes should have their interests safeguarded by the law, which ensures that the people owning and running homes are in all respects fit to do so, and that they provide accommodation, facilities, and amenities that are adequate for the comfort, dignity, and enjoyment of life of those who live there.

It also means that if a resident in a home is not satisfied with the conditions there, and complaints to the management have not resulted in any improvements, there is a higher authority to whom he can take his complaint: the registering authority, whose inspector should investigate it and see that things are put right. The government intend to require a notice to be placed in homes explaining how a complaint can be made.

Mary Hughes, a widow of 78, went into a private rest home some years after her husband died, after she had had a very bad fall and broken her leg, which left her lame. She also began to get rather forgetful, and her married son urged her to go into a home where she could be properly looked after. She would much rather have stayed in her own home, but to please her son she agreed. The home seemed quite nice at first, and it was a relief not having to do housework or cook her own meals, but she took badly to having to share a room with a stranger, and asked to be moved to a single room as soon as one fell vacant. In the meantime, she found there was nowhere to lock her valuable possessions away in safety, nor could she lock her door if she wanted to be on her own. Because she shared, she couldn't use her room as a sitting-room, and there was nowhere private to take visitors when they came to see her. In addition to this, she found there were very rigid rules about the times for getting up and going to bed, as well as for meals to be served, and she had to let a member of staff know whenever she left the home for any reason. Her pension book had been taken away from her, and the manager of the home doled out her 'pocket money' once a week. Altogether she felt as though she was living in an institution like the old workhouse, and she became very unhappy.

One day when her son was visiting her she poured all her troubles out to him, and he was so shocked that he went straight to the manager of the home to complain at the way his mother and other residents were being treated. The woman in charge – who both owned and managed the home – was very offhand and unhelpful, but reluctantly said she would see what could be done to improve life for Mary. However, there was not only no change for the better, but a distinct change for the worse, as the manager kept making unpleasant, sarcastic remarks to Mary about her being ungrateful, and a 'moaning Minnie', and what a silly, forgetful old woman she was. Mary burst into tears on her son's shoulder the next time he came; he couldn't take her home with him because there wasn't enough room in his small house for her, but he promised he would look around for another home for her, and in the meantime decided to report this home to the local social services department and ask them if they could do anything to improve it. They listened to him sympathetically, and sent an inspector round within a few days, who checked on all the things Mary found so difficult and irksome. The manager was then told that if she didn't relax her rules and regulations and make life much more pleasant and normal for her residents, they would have to consider cancelling her registration. Shocked at the idea of losing her livelihood, she obeyed his instructions, and even began to treat Mary with respect. But fortunately her son found another home with a much more pleasant and homely atmosphere, where Mary could have her own room, her treasured possessions around her, come and go as she pleased, and be surrounded by warmth and kindness.

Are there any other safeguards?

There are three other organisations which try to ensure that standards in homes are high: these are the Registered Nursing Home Association (RNHA), the National Confederation of Registered Rest Homes Associations (NCRRHA), and the British Federation of Care-Home Proprietors (BFCHP). The RNHA represents nursing home owners, and the other two organisations represent residential care home owners. These organisations were formed because of concern among home-owners that the private sector was getting a bad reputation for poor standards and exploitation of residents. They wanted to restore the balance, raise standards, and demonstrate that privately owned homes can and do play a valuable part in providing a service to dependent elderly people.

All three organisations insist on high standards among their members, and are concerned that staff employed in homes should be properly trained. They support the concept of registration, and work closely with their respective registering authorities to see that high standards are maintained. They have their own inspection systems to complement those operated by the health and local authorities.

Each organisation has its own symbol which members can display. The RNHA uses a distinctive blue cross, the NCRRHA a clever design of a house made up from its initials, and the BFCHP displays two caring hands enclosing the figures of two frail people. So if you see these symbols on the door-plate of a home, you will know that the owner is a member of the association and the home ought to have a good standard of care to offer.

RNHA

BFCHP

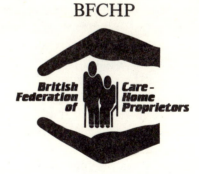

NCRRHA

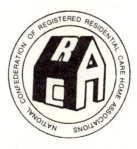

Who inspects?

There is a very serious weakness, however, in the new legislation governing residential care homes. The inspectors do not have responsibility for inspecting local authority homes as well as those that are privately owned. Even if they did, they would be open to accusations of bias, since inspecting teams consist of staff from the local authority social service departments. Everyone who has been horrified by the reports of the callous and cruel treatment alleged to have been meted out to elderly residents by some 'care' staff at a local authority home in a London borough, will wonder how such treatment could go unnoticed and unchecked by those in charge of and responsible for the home. What standards would an authority which allows this to happen in one of its own homes, apply to privately owned homes in its area?

The simple and obvious solution to this very serious problem is to set up inspectorates which are independent of local (or health) authorities, and which are responsible for inspecting all types of home, applying the same standards to local authority, private, and voluntary or charitable homes. Such inspectorates would apply compulsory guidelines for standards of care, and have the power to cancel registrations if standards fall below an acceptable level.

The 1984 Act is obviously not working as well as it should be if cases of cruelty to and intimidation of elderly residents in care are still being revealed, so the Government should act quickly to prevent this continuing by revising the legislation accordingly: by setting up independent inspectorates, and making codes of practice compulsory and universal.

Chapter six

What are my rights as a resident in a rest home?

Dorothy Smith lived in a small rest home run by a charitable organisation. There were only six other residents, most of them women, and each had a room of her own, with a wash-hand basin, and they were allowed to have some of their own furniture as well. Dorothy had her own television set, so that she could watch her favourite programmes when she wanted to. There was a bathroom and separate toilet near her room, and a kitchenette on the same floor where she could make a cup of tea for herself or for her visitors if she wanted to. The lounge and dining-room were pleasant and comfortable; there was a nice garden, too, where Dorothy – who had a passion for gardening – could lend a hand when she felt like it, and cut some flowers to decorate her room. The staff were all polite and friendly; nothing was too much trouble, and Dorothy felt really happy and 'at home'.

Dorothy's friend Betty Jones had gone to live in a larger home nearby when her husband died, but she wasn't nearly so happy. To begin with, she had to share a room, and although she tried hard, she couldn't get on with her room-mate, whose habits she found very irritating. She couldn't use her room as a sitting-room, and had to be out of it soon after breakfast so that the staff could clean it. The lounge was always full, everyone had their favourite chairs so that she had to take whatever was left, and the television set was on all day, much too loud to permit conversation. There were strict rules about meal-times, having visitors, and using the telephone, and the staff were offhand and familiar, and always in too much of a hurry to stop for a pleasant chat. She hated being called 'Gran' or 'dearie', as they never used her proper name, and she felt that she had completely lost her own identity and position in the world.

'It's just like being in the workhouse', Betty used to say to Dorothy when they met, as they did regularly, at the local cafe for a cup of tea. 'I wish I could move into your home – or at least do something to improve matters in my home. But the woman in charge doesn't like people complaining. She gets very impatient and rude, so it's simply not worth the trouble she would make.'

It was to help people like Betty that, when the Registered Homes Act 1984 was in its preliminary stages, the Secretary of State for Social Services asked the Centre for Policy on Ageing (CPA) to produce a code of practice for home owners and managers. This code, entitled *Home Life*, was published in 1984, and is intended to be used as a guideline for good practice by both the authorities which register and inspect rest homes, and by the proprietors and managers of these homes. It sets out clearly what rights the residents of rest homes should expect to have, and what sort of care and consideration they are entitled to be given.

It is another weakness of the Act that it did not make this code of practice mandatory: that is to say, it does not *have* to be followed, but is intended to provide local authorities with a basis for the guidelines to practice which each one is entitled to prepare for use in its own area. It is a greater weakness that the code of practice is not enforced on local authority homes as well, and that these homes are not subject to the same regulations regarding inspections as are private homes. Each local authority social services department should apply the same strict standards to its own homes as to privately owned homes registered with it.

The rights of residents

The rights of residents in rest homes are given pride of place in this code of practice which states categorically that all who live in residential care should be able to do so with dignity; they should have the respect of those who support them; their rights as citizens should not be reduced; and they should be entitled to live as full and active a life as their physical and mental condition will allow. This means that rest home owners and managers should do all they can to enable their residents to live the sort of lives they would in their own homes, with as much privacy, freedom, and independence as is possible in a communal home.

This may sound fine in theory, but how can it be achieved in practice? The code lists a number of principles of care, some very practical, like the right to a single room, and some more abstract, which are concerned with what is often called the QUALITY OF LIFE. The first of these abstract principles is FULFILMENT: the right to lead the sort of life which satisfies a resident as an individual. The second is DIGNITY: the right to personal privacy, and to be treated at all times with courtesy and respect. This includes the right to one's own beliefs and opinions, and to express them or to keep them to oneself, as one wishes.

Third comes AUTONOMY – the right not to be regimented, or live to a strict routine, but to do what one wants to do when one wants to do it, provided that one abides by the rules that all communities, large and small, must lay down so that the communal existence is peaceful, secure, and well ordered, and individuals do not infringe each others' rights.

INDIVIDUALITY is the fourth right, or principle of care. This is especially important for elderly people from other countries and races who have made their homes in Britain and have now reached the time of life when they need more care and support.

As residents they should have the right to follow their own religion, customs, dress, and diet, for example. But for everyone, irrespective of race, it is important to be able to preserve one's individuality, to follow one's own tastes and preferences in all sorts of ways, and the code says this right should be respected in rest homes.

Old people are too often nowadays regarded as a nuisance, a burden, and treated as though their years of experience and achievement, and the wisdom derived from them, count for nothing. They are accorded little, if any, esteem – and ESTEEM is the fifth right listed in this code: a 'knowledge and respect for the individual's life history', and 'a positive regard for family and friends, where they exist'.

QUALITY OF EXPERIENCE is another right, and this includes such material benefits as having your own possessions around you, being able to go shopping, to church, to the cinema, theatre, pub, clubs, or to follow any other pursuit you may enjoy or find satisfying. Emotional needs are also important, and the development of personal relationships should be the right of residents. There is no reason why older people should not find happiness and affection in close companionship with each other, and marriage is by no means an unknown event in these circumstances.

Last but not least is the right to take RESPONSIBLE RISKS. It is a temptation to protect a vulnerable person from accident or injury by limiting his freedom to go out and about by himself, but this is the easy way out and not kind. It is far better to allow an elderly person to decide for himself whether or not, if he wants to do something where risk is involved, that risk is worth taking, provided of course that other people are not also put at risk, or caused a lot of trouble.

These rights are intangible, and concern people's attitudes towards the elderly and towards those, in particular, who have to surrender the freedom of life in their own homes for the more secure surroundings of a rest home. They are very important, and all good home owners and managers should observe them punctiliously.

Practical rights

There are other, more tangible, rights that a prospective resident of a rest home should expect, and life will be easier if you can find out if they are respected before you go into the home.

First and foremost, you should expect to be given FULL AND ACCURATE INFORMATION ABOUT THE HOME, in the form of a brochure setting out details of the accommodation offered, the terms and conditions, the staff employed, and the facilities available. It should make clear what you are paying for and what, if anything, you will be charged for as an extra. It should be possible for you to visit the home before making the decision to go into it, and also for the home owner or manager to visit you so that you can get to know each other better, if you would like that.

Most important is the right, once the decision has been made, to stay in the home for a TRIAL PERIOD of, say, two or three months, so that if you shouldn't like it for any reason, you can change your mind and go back to your own home while you look for another one. Do not on any account sell your home or end your tenancy until this trial period is over and you are as certain as you can be that you want to stay. This trial period, incidentally, gives the proprietor a chance to make sure that you fit in with the other residents too!

Rules and regulations

Every home is bound to have some rules and regulations so that it can be run smoothly, and the interests of all the residents be catered for. For example, smoking can be a pleasure to some and an offence to others, so there should be rules about where smoking is permitted and where it is not. Rules to beware of are those which are solely in the interests of the home, and bear no relevance to the well-being of residents.

But there should be as few rules as possible, and residents should be consulted and their opinions taken into account when new rules are made, or existing rules changed. Residents should, indeed, have the opportunity to be involved in the running of the home, either as individuals or through a residents' committee.

Complaints

Older people are usually reluctant to complain when things are not to their liking, because they don't want to make a fuss or be regarded as trouble-makers. It is even more difficult when you are dependent on someone you may wish to complain about. It is important, however, that a resident should be able to complain about something he finds unsatisfactory without fear that his complaint will either be brushed aside or dismissed as unimportant, or rebound on him in the form of unpleasant behaviour or even the threat of eviction from the home.

This code states that it is the right of residents to complain about any matter, but particularly about infringements of the code itself, and to have their complaints treated seriously and recorded. If matters are not put right, or if the resident feels that he is being victimised by the head or proprietor of the home, he can take his complaint to the registering authority. If he doesn't want to do this himself, someone can do it on his behalf. The government intends that a notice explaining the complaint procedure shall be displayed in every home.

If a resident is worried that he may be turned out of a home, and is not sure what his rights are, he should consult the Citizen's Advice Bureau or local law centre, or branch of the Law Society, to find a solicitor to give him legal advice. It's worth remembering that residents cannot normally be evicted from a home without a Court order.

Privacy and autonomy

One of the most worrying things about the prospect of going into a home must be the thought of losing one's personal freedom and privacy. The code recognises this very real anxiety, and strongly recommends that all residents in rest homes should have their own rooms (unless they prefer to share) where they can lock the door if they want to be private, and where they can have a reasonable amount of their own furniture and personal possessions around them. Residents should be allowed to look after their own rooms, and staff should only enter with their permission. For safety's sake, of course, each room should have an alarm call system, and there should be a master key so that staff can get into all rooms in cases of emergency.

The code goes into detail about such necessities as furniture and storage and hanging space, and emphasises that all residents should be able to wash, dress, and use the toilet in private. You should also be able to see whom you like in a private sitting-room, and have access to the telephone. You should also have the right to take your personal possessions into the rest home – or as many as there are room for – and to have them treated with care and respect by the staff. You should always be able to wear your own clothes, and never have to wear any from a common pool of clothing.

The freedom to go out and about – on shopping expeditions, for walks, to the public library, or simply to meet friends – is also regarded as important, though the code sensibly says that as a matter of courtesy residents should let staff know their whereabouts if they are going out, and when they are likely to return. Caring staff will naturally worry about a resident who is absent for a long time if they don't know where he or she is. Longer visits to family and friends should be encouraged, as well as holidays away from the home. Equally, friends and relatives should be encouraged to visit residents, and to keep in touch by letter and telephone.

If a resident has no family or friends, the home staff should encourage voluntary helpers to make contact and see if there is any way in which they can be of help – perhaps by inviting them to visit their own homes, to do little chores like shopping and letter writing, or just by sitting and talking. Some Age Concern groups organise such a service.

It can be very irritating, and even humiliating, to be called by your first name or by a nickname, or just 'Gran' or 'Dad' or 'dearie' or 'ducks', by someone you don't know or who is there to look after you. Under this code it is a resident's right to be addressed by his proper name and title (ie Mr, Mrs, Ms or Miss Smith) by all staff unless they have his permission to address him informally.

Financial affairs

Whatever age you may be, and if you own any property at all, it is a wise precaution to make a will, so that if you should die suddenly or unexpectedly your affairs will be in order and your money and possessions will go to people you want to have them. If and when you go into a residential home, you should make a will before you move, but if you leave it until you have moved in, the code points out that it should be done independently of the proprietor or staff of the home. You should not, for instance, use the proprietor's solicitor, or ask him or any member of the staff to act as witness or to be an executor. A good home proprietor will also want to avoid this. If you have no family solicitor, you should find one through the Law Society or the local Citizen's Advice Bureau. The code says that, ideally, home owners should not allow residents to give presents or tips to staff, other than small 'token' gifts.

Incidents have been reported in the press of home owners or managers taking control of their residents' money and pension books. The code of practice states categorically that residents must be responsible for their own money, valuables, pension books, and other documents, and that the home must supply a safe or lockable cupboard where they can be deposited. A careful record of all deposits must be kept by the home management and receipts be given for all items deposited, so that there is no possibility of them 'going astray'.

If you become frail

A person who is very frail or has poor sight or hearing, for instance, may need someone to act for him – to draw his pension, cash cheques, pay bills and so on. If there is no relative or friend to do this, the local social services department should be asked to find someone suitable or trustworthy – or, if you don't want to be involved with the social services, you could approach a voluntary group such as Age Concern. The owner or manager of the home should not be asked to take over unless it is absolutely impossible to find someone else.

If there is a lot of personal business to be handled, it may be necessary to give someone the power of attorney, or to set up a trust, and in these circumstances a solicitor should always be consulted; no one connected with the home should be involved. It might be preferable to take out an enduring power of attorney which would last even if the person is no longer able to handle his own affairs. The Court of Protection provides an informative leaflet about powers of attorney for those considering this possibility.

Sadly, our mental powers sometimes deteriorate with age, so that we may become unable to think for ourselves and make decisions. Then the local social services department should be asked to find someone suitable to act for us, but it should never be the manager or proprietor of the home. A resident in this state of mental confusion who is well off, or has a lot of assets to be managed, should be placed under the jurisdiction of the Court of Protection. An application to the Court can be made by a relative, friend, social worker, or indeed anyone, but it must be accompanied by a medical certificate from the resident's GP explaining why it is necessary. If the Court accepts the application, it will appoint a 'receiver' to manage that resident's affairs, who is often a relative – but, again, in no circumstances should the receiver be connected with the home.

This part of the code is designed to protect residents from being financially exploited, and home owners and managers from being laid open to accusations of misconduct of residents' affairs. It is a very wise safeguard for both parties.

Keeping healthy

Your health is particularly important to you at this time of your life, and although some disability may have forced you into looking for a place in a rest home, you will still want to remain as fit and active as possible. The head of the home will need to know the details of your medical condition and of any treatment you may be having, but these details should only be given with your consent, and should be treated in the strictest confidence. You will not have to give up your own family doctor if the rest home is within his practice area; if not, you can still choose your own GP from those practising in the home's locality. You need not go on the list of the home's doctor unless you choose to.

If you should fall ill and need skilled nursing for a short period, the district nurse will call just as she would in your own home, and the routine care which a relative would normally give you will be carried out by the staff of the home. If your illness is protracted so that you require continual skilled nursing, you may have to move into a nursing home. If you are lucky enough to find a home with dual registration as both rest home and nursing home, you can be nursed in your own familiar surroundings.

You may need to take certain medicines for a permanent condition such as diabetes, rheumatoid arthritis, or high blood pressure, and the home should encourage you to be responsible for taking your own drugs for as long as you are able to do so, and should provide a drawer or cupboard which can be locked for you to keep them in. If for any reason – such as poor sight – you cannot take your own drugs, the proprietor of the home should see they are kept in a safe place, clearly labelled with your name and the dosage you should have, and that they are given to you at the right time by someone who is trained and authorised to do so. Careful records should also be kept of all drugs prescribed for and given to residents.

When you reach the end of your life, you have the right to be cared for in a rest home just as you would be at home – peacefully in your own bed, attended by your own doctor, with your family and friends round you, and with skilled district nurses coming in to care for you. You should be reassured that, whatever your race and religious faith, your spiritual needs will be attended to and, when the time comes, your funeral will be conducted as you would wish it to be. However, not all rest homes are willing to look after people right up to the end of their lives, so this is something to ask about when you are searching for the right one.

Home Life is very comprehensive, and has proved so successful that it has recently been translated into Japanese! It is an excellent guide to the rights you should have as a resident in a rest home. And don't forget that it is intended to be observed by rest home proprietors and managers, and that if it is infringed in any way, residents have just cause for complaint. Remember, though, that it may have been adapted by the local authority in your area to form the basis of its own guidelines; if so, it is worth asking them for a copy. They should apply, incidentally, to local authority Part III homes just as much as to privately owned or voluntary homes.

Chapter seven
What are my rights as a resident in a nursing home?

John Wilkinson, who was aged 75, had developed Parkinson's disease soon after he turned 70. At first his doctor managed to control his symptoms with the drug L-dopa, but after a couple of years it began to lose its effect, and John found his symptoms getting worse. His hands shook, he found walking difficult, he had several bad falls because he couldn't keep his balance, and finally his speech became affected – he couldn't form his words.

This was very distressing both for John and his wife Susan, who looked after him devotedly in spite of the fact that her joints were very painful from rheumatism, and she found handling him and getting about quite a problem. John worried about his wife and about the future, because he knew he was becoming a burden to her which might one day be intolerable, and this made his own symptoms worse.

One day their family doctor, who could see what was happening, talked to them seriously about the future and said he thought the time had come when caring for John was getting too much for Susan, and they should think about the possibility of his going into a nursing home, as it was unlikely his condition would improve. There were a number of homes in the district which provided skilled nursing care, and as John had a good pension from his job in the insurance business, and had also saved carefully during his working life, he could afford the fees for the time being, at any rate. So Susan went to the local Citizen's Advice Bureau, which gave her a list of nursing homes in the area and suggested she visit those whose fees they could afford.

Susan went to see as many as she could, but she found it difficult to know what to look for, and how to judge whether a home was good or not, so eventually she chose the one nearest to their own home, so that she could visit John easily and often. It was quite a large nursing home, owned by a private company; it seemed clean and well-appointed, and when the Matron said there was a small room vacant on the top floor at a reasonable charge, Susan decided to reserve it for John. The room was at the back of the building overlooking a busy road. It was certainly small, with the minimum of furniture in it, but the Matron said a larger, more comfortable room would probably fall free soon which John could have if he wanted it.

John moved in at the end of the week, and at first everything seemed fine. He found it a relief to have trained nurses looking after him: they knew what his needs were, and he didn't have to worry about being too much trouble to them. But then a number of little things began to irk him. The food wasn't very good, to begin with, and nobody helped him eat although he had trouble with chewing and swallowing his meals. Then he found that the nurses, although they seemed brisk and efficient, didn't show much sympathy or understanding, or take an interest in him as a person; he felt they regarded him as just another 'poor old thing' who was a bit of a nuisance. Some of them got quite irritable if he was incontinent and soiled the bed, which he couldn't help doing during the night. Also the toilet was at the other end of the corridor from his room, and sometimes he couldn't reach it in time, which he found very upsetting.

Then, except for Susan's visits, he found he got very bored and lonely as there was very little to do all day except read or watch television. There was no communal lounge, and the nursing home didn't provide any recreational or social events. All the other patients seemed to keep to their rooms, except one on his floor who became a positive menace. He was an elderly man who was obviously very confused, and would wander along the corridor at all hours of the day and night, sometimes shouting aggressively, and going into the other rooms and disturbing the occupants. The nurses did very little to try and control him; they gave John the impression they thought he was making a fuss when he tried to complain.

As John's speech got worse he found it more and more difficult to communicate with the nursing home staff, none of whom took the time to talk to him or help him to talk to them. The staff changed constantly in any case; a lot of the nurses came from agencies and only worked at the home for a few weeks before moving on, so they didn't bother to get to know the patients. Altogether, he began to feel desperately unhappy, and although he tried to put a brave face on it for his wife, one day he found himself pouring out his troubles to her – she was the only person who could understand him.

Susan was horrified, and decided there and then to take him back home with her, no matter how difficult it would be to look after him. She rang their doctor to tell him what had happened; he came to see them the next day, and arranged for the district nurse to visit every day while they decided what to do next.

By good fortune, the district nurse was a very kindly, experienced woman who at one time had worked in a hospital geriatric unit, and taken a special training course in the care of the elderly. She recognised John's special needs, and obtained from the health authority a list of nursing homes in the district on which her nursing colleagues at the health authority indicated those which they thought would suit. One of these homes looked very promising. It was owned and managed by a nurse who had recently left the National Health Service to operate her own nursing home with the aim of providing first-class nursing care to older people. Although the home was further away than the one John had left, Susan got in touch with the owner to find out if she had a vacancy. The owner said there was a room falling vacant soon, and invited Susan over to see it.

This nursing home was in a large old house with attractive grounds, specially converted for the purpose. It took only twelve patients, each of whom had a spacious single room with toilet and washing facilities, and a pleasant outlook over the gardens. There was a pleasant, well-furnished lounge and dining room; a small sitting-room for visitors; and the whole atmosphere was relaxed and friendly, more like a small country hotel than a place for sick people. All the staff had special training in caring for the elderly, and their attitude was courteous and helpful.

Susan was very impressed with all she saw, and by the difference between this small, homely establishment and the other, larger and much more impersonal nursing home. She liked the owner, Mrs Brown, who also acted as Matron: she combined authority and efficiency with warmth and friendly understanding, and Susan felt instinctively this was someone whom she could trust with John's welfare. The residents to whom Susan spoke were all relaxed and friendly as well, and obviously contented with their care.

Two weeks later Mrs Brown telephoned to say the room was now free if John wanted it; Susan had no hesitation in accepting it, and moved John in. He settled down quickly and comfortably, and Susan knew that he would be well cared for at last.

Making a good choice

This case history illustrates the difference there can be between two nursing homes in the same area, and how difficult it can be to know how to choose one that provides the quality of care you are looking for. There are of course good and bad nursing homes – but if you know what you are entitled to expect from them, you are more likely to make a good choice.

When the Registered Homes Act 1984 was still a bill going through Parliament, the Secretary of State for Social Services asked an organisation called the National Association of Health Authorities (NAHA) to prepare guidelines on the registration and inspection of private hospitals and nursing homes. These guidelines were published in January 1985 (when the Act came into force) as a *Handbook for Health Authorities*, a comprehensive guide to the kind of care and standards required in private nursing homes, for use both by the health authorities responsible for registration and inspection and persons in charge of private nursing homes and hospitals.

This guide was intended to be used as a basis for the guidelines each health authority prepared for its individual purpose, and although – like the code of practice for residential care – it was not compulsory under the Act, it was hoped that it would be widely followed and set a high national standard.

Quality of care

The overall aim of the guidelines is to ensure that the quality of care provided to patients in private nursing homes is good. They should be able to live in comfortable, clean, and safe surroundings, and be treated with respect and sensitivity to their individual needs and abilities. The special needs of elderly people are considered, the governing factor being the degree to which they are dependent on others for their daily needs.

The guidelines stress that nursing homes should be organised and the staff motivated to give patients the greatest degree of independence possible, and also that they should have plenty of recreation – opportunities to occupy both their time and their minds with things they enjoy. Maintaining dignity and privacy are also regarded as very important.

Information

The first thing that a potential resident in a nursing home needs is information about the home itself: the accommodation, facilities, and services it offers; the fees it charges; the staffing levels, and so on. The guide therefore specifies that every nursing home should provide a brochure giving all these details for potential residents, their families and friends who may be acting on their behalf.

Every private nursing home must also be registered under the Act, and display a certificate of registration from the health authority in a prominent position. It is an offence against the law to carry on a nursing home without being registered, and not to display this certificate.

Staff

The home must employ people who are properly trained and qualified, and it is up to the person in charge – who must be a qualified doctor or nurse – to check the qualifications of all its staff. This is to ensure that patients are efficiently nursed by competent staff during both day and night. The person in charge must also see that there is someone sufficiently experienced and responsible to deputise for him or her in periods of absence, and that there are qualified nurses on duty at all times who will supervise nursing auxiliaries and other untrained or temporary staff.

If other professional staff, such as physiotherapists, occupational therapists, chiropodists, and speech therapists, are employed, their qualifications must also be checked. Catering and domestic staff, too, must be adequately experienced and provide a high standard of hygiene and cleanliness.

Patients are, of course, entitled to be under the medical care of their own GPs, and if a specialist opinion is needed, the GP should arrange for an appropriate specialist to visit.

Accommodation

The guidelines go on to say that nursing homes should be located away from noise, heavy traffic, smells, and 'environmental pollution', and that they should be kept in a good state of repair and decoration.

There must be adequate bathrooms and lavatories, which should be equipped with grab rails and have non-slip flooring. Doors should be wide enough to admit a wheelchair, and there should be room for hoists to help disabled patients get in and out of the bath.

There should be toilets on each floor, with facilities for washing hands.

Complaints

After dealing with required standards for heating, lighting, and ventilation, furniture and equipment, size and type of accommodation, food service, linen and laundry, waste disposal, infection control, control of drugs and other medicines, fire safety, accident prevention, and record keeping, the guidelines cover the important subject of complaints, saying that they should be dealt with quickly and effectively by those in charge, and justified grievances promptly remedied.

Under the Act's Regulations, an authorised person must be able to interview any patient in private. This means that the patient must have the opportunity to speak freely, without being inhibited by the presence of a third party – possibly a member of the nursing home staff.

Complaints about the professional conduct of doctors and nurses should, if they cannot be resolved, be referred to the General Medical Council (in the case of doctors), or to the UK Central Council for Nursing, Midwifery, and Health Visiting or to the appropriate National Board for Nursing (in the case of nurses). The addresses of these bodies are in the 'Useful Organisations' section at the back of this book.

If the patient is occupying a nursing home bed which is subsidised by the DHSS, the same complaints procedure should be followed as in the NHS: that is to say, it should be made to the District Health Authority; or, if it concerns the patient's GP, to the local Family Practitioner Committee.

If help or advice is needed in making a complaint, it is always worth contacting the local Community Health Council, which has a sort of 'watchdog' function on local health services, and can offer guidance in instances where nursing home places are under contract from NHS hospitals; or the local branch of Age Concern.

Special needs

A section of these model guidelines is devoted to the special needs of older people. This section emphasises that staff should be flexible in their approach and sensitive to the changing needs of each patient. They should always be helping them to be independent, and giving them plenty with which to occupy their time: not just entertainment or social activity, but something useful and interesting to do, as older people like to feel that they can still be useful.

Nursing homes for the elderly should be clean, comfortable, safe, and domestic in character rather than coldly clinical, and patients should at all times be able to retain their dignity and privacy. They should be encouraged to bring their personal possessions, including furniture, into the home, and there should be plenty of storage space for their belongings. There should also be pleasant rooms where they can spend their time during the day. All steps and stairs should have handrails and be properly carpeted, to prevent patients from tripping and falling.

One of the most distressing and humiliating conditions that older people have to endure is incontinence, so quick and easy access to a toilet is vital, and can help to avoid 'accidents'. The guidelines stress this important point, and also say there should be adequate laundry facilities and ventilation, to avoid unpleasant smells. Also all bathrooms and toilets or other places where patients may have to undress should be properly heated.

Furnishing

How a nursing home is furnished can make all the difference to an older person's safety and comfort. For instance, any carpeting should be 'wall to wall' so that there is no danger of tripping over loose rugs. Large patterns on floor coverings should also be avoided as someone with poor sight might easily mistake the pattern for an obstacle.

Also, all furnishing should be of a material that can be cleaned quickly and easily, to prevent unpleasant smells or stains that hang around. Bedrooms should have proper dressing-tables and wardrobes, and enough cupboards in which to keep personal belongings or materials used for hobbies. Chairs should be carefully chosen to suit each individual, as a comfortable chair that provides good support and is easy to get into and out of is essential.

The patient's day

The way you spend your day can also make all the difference to your life: an older person doesn't want to be regimented, and does want to keep active and interested. The model guidelines say that the elderly patient's day should not be rigidly organised. They should not, for instance, be wakened too early in the morning, just to suit the nurses, and they should be allowed to decide for themselves when to go to bed. They should be able to go out and about as freely as their physical condition permits, and outings and shopping expeditions should be arranged for them.

Last, but certainly by no means least, visiting hours in nursing homes should be as free and flexible as possible.

To sum up

You will see from reading this that the guidelines prepared by NAHA are a model of the care that all private nursing homes should provide. However, as they are not compulsory, it is inevitable that standards still vary from one district to another and from one home to another.

However, now that you know what you are entitled to expect, it should be easier for you to judge a good nursing home from a bad one. And don't forget that, where private homes are concerned, he who pays the piper should be able to call the tune!

Chapter eight
How do I go about finding a home?

Before you actually start looking for a home, you must be sure in your own mind that this is the right move for you. You mustn't allow yourself to be influenced or pressurised by other people, no matter how good their intentions may be. The decision must be yours and yours alone, in the end, and it must only be taken after a lot of careful thought.

Having decided to take this important step, you must then make sure it is not irrevocable. That is to say, having found a home which seems suitable, you must not on any account burn your boats by selling your house, or giving notice to quit if your dwelling is rented, before you have stayed in the home for a trial period to see if it really does suit you. If it proves unsatisfactory for some reason or other, you must be able to return to your own home while you look around for another one – or even decide not to go into a home after all.

Hospitals are always under pressure with waiting lists for beds, and a consultant may decide to discharge a patient who, in his opinion, does not need more medical treatment, even though he or she may have been in hospital for some time and still need nursing care. In such a situation, you or your relatives acting for you should ask the hospital social worker for help in finding a suitable rest home or nursing home, and for advice on applying for financial assistance towards the cost. You should also ask the consultant in charge of your case for sufficient time to visit homes before selecting one, so that you are not pressurised into making the move too quickly and without enough consideration.

A good hospital will take a lot of trouble to assess your particular needs so that they can advise you about the type of home and facilities to look for. This may mean that the doctors, nurses, social workers, and others may ask you all sorts of questions about both your physical condition and your domestic circumstances. This process is called 'assessment', and its purpose is to help you to find a home in which you will be properly looked after and have your special requirements catered for. The practice of assessing older patients before they leave hospital is not yet universal by any means, but specialists in geriatric medicine are trying to encourage their colleagues to do this for the benefit of their patients.

Where?

Having made your decision, the first thing to consider is the location. It is important to bear in mind that you will want to be near your family and friends, so that they can come and visit you frequently and you can go and see them. Even if you have difficulty in getting around, it is good to get out and about and see people once in a while. You are bound to feel lonely in the first weeks after moving in, and that is when you will need them most, before you have had a chance to make new friends in the home. So try to stay in your familiar neighbourhood, near your friends, or to find a home near your relatives if they live some distance away from you. But be sure your family really will visit you regularly and give you support and companionship, and not leave you feeling deserted in unfamiliar surroundings.

The next thing is to contact your local social services department for help and advice. Your options will be either to go into a local authority home, or into one that is privately owned, or run by a charitable organisation. The social worker on duty should explain to you – or your relative, if one is acting on your behalf – what local authority homes there are in your neighbourhood, how to go about applying for a place in one, what the procedure will be, and how much you are likely to be charged. The next chapter goes into the whole question of fees and what help you can get towards them if you need it.

Local authority homes

If you do choose to go into a local authority home, you may find that there is a long waiting list for places. The support of your family doctor in your application might help to give you priority, if your case is urgent. A social worker will visit you to find out more about your particular needs, and he or she will give you a list of the homes in your district, and either take you to visit them or ask the head of the home to arrange this. Then when you have seen them all, and chosen which one you prefer, and the financial arrangements have been agreed, you should be able to stay in the home for a trial period of about three months, at the end of which you can decide if you want to become a permanent resident there. It is worth bearing in mind, however, that if you decide against one home where you are offered a place, you may have a long wait before you are offered a place in another home.

Your individual needs, circumstances, and wishes will be reviewed by the social services staff at regular intervals during your trial stay, and if you do become a permanent resident, to make sure it is the right place for you. They should have your overall welfare at heart.

If you want to move outside your county to be near a relative, you will of course come under a different local authority. Each local authority makes its own conditions for residents in its care homes, so they may be different in the area you want to move to. There is usually a condition giving priority to applicants who have lived in the area for some time. It is wise to consult your own local social services department first, who will be able to give you any information and advice you need, as these departments do keep in touch with each other, and you will need the support of your own local authority, particularly if you cannot afford the full fees.

It is also worth remembering that local authority homes quite often accept residents for short periods – in an emergency, for instance, or when a relative caring for someone needs a break or a holiday. This is known as 'respite care', and can be arranged by the local social services department.

Private or voluntary homes

You may, however, decide that you would prefer to look for a private home, or one run by a voluntary charitable organisation. Here again your first point of contact is your local social services department. The social worker on duty may pass you on to the person with special responsibility for residential care, who should give you a list of the private and voluntary rest and nursing homes in the district, together with the names and addresses of the homes and their owners, and the fees they charge. You or your relative will be recommended to go and visit those which are in the right area and within your income. It is worth remembering that it is possible to get financial help from the DHSS towards paying the fees, as you will read in the next chapter.

Your local Citizen's Advice Bureau and your local Age Concern group should also be useful sources of information and advice. Many of them keep lists of homes in their areas, together with details of their charges and the type of accommodation they offer. The CAB is a voluntary organisation which exists to provide, free of charge to all individuals, an impartial service of information, guidance, and support.

If you live in London or the south of England there are two organisations which specifically help elderly people to find suitable residential care or nursing homes: they are Counsel and Care for the Elderly (CCE); and GRACE, Mrs Gould's Residential Advisory Centre for the Elderly. CCE has a team of case workers who visit all the registered private and voluntary homes in the Greater London area annually, in order to be able to give advice to those looking for a home. The team also provides an information and counselling service, which is free and confidential, to individual enquiries relating to homes and housing, financial assistance for nursing care at home and in residential accommodation, holidays, statutory benefits, help with bills, temporary care to give relatives a break, and lump sum grants for specific needs.

GRACE also compiles detailed information about privately owned residential care and nursing homes, and offers advice about accommodation to suit individual needs. The service covers the 25 counties in the south of England, and a registration fee is charged (currently £15) which is returnable when a client becomes a resident in a home recommended by GRACE.

You may also find it useful to go to the reference section in your local public library, where you should find such directories as the *Charities Digest*, and the *Directory of Private Hospitals and Health Services* (both these publications are listed at the back of this book). The *Charities Digest* gives details of all charitable organisations, listed alphabetically. It uses a code of letters to signify which are concerned with providing housing and residential care for elderly people. The *Directory of Private Hospitals and Health Services* lists the names, addresses, and phone numbers of, as well as some details about, private nursing homes and residential care homes.

The Registered Nursing Home Association publishes a reference book of registered nursing homes, clinics, and hospitals in the UK; and Croner Publications have also published a directory of residential care homes. See also Age Concern England Factsheet No. 29, "Finding Residential and Nursing Home Accommodation".

Your check-list

Now you come to the stage of visiting those homes in your area of choice which look promising, and it is as well to prepare yourself by making a list of things to check as you are shown over the home, and questions to ask about it. Then when you have visited several, you can compare the answers to your questions in each case and see which one comes out best.

- First, and most important, is it registered, and does it have a certificate of registration displayed conspicuously in the entrance hall? Is it also in membership with the National Confederation of Registered Residential Care Homes Associations, displaying its symbol of a small house; with the British Federation of Care Home Proprietors, displaying its symbol of the caring hands; or with the Registered Nursing Home Association, displaying a Blue Cross symbol? All these organisations should ensure that homes owned by members maintain a good standard of care.

- Are you given a brochure providing all the factual information you need about the home, such as the number and size of the rooms, the services provided, and the scale of charges, as well as a list of additional charges not included in the fees?

- Is the home for both sexes, or for one sex only?

- How near is it to your family and friends, and is public transport easily accessible? Is there a shopping centre nearby?

- Are there plenty of single rooms, some with their own bathrooms, shower rooms, or toilet, but all with wash-hand basins? Are the double rooms reserved only for married couples or close friends wishing to share, or would you be expected to share with a total stranger? Are there any rooms where more than two people are expected to share? (If so, this home is not obeying the code of practice.)

- Are there plenty of bathrooms and separate toilets, and are they easy to reach? Are they equipped with lever-handled taps, grab rails, and raised toilet seats, and are the doors wide enough for a wheelchair or a walking aid to pass through? Are there aids to help you get on and off the toilet, and into and out of the bath?

- Are there alarm call systems in every room?

- Are there telephones in residents' rooms? If not, may they have them installed if they want one? Is there a public telephone within easy access on each floor if personal telephones are not available?

- Are residents allowed to bring their own furniture and possessions into the home, or are there any restrictions?

- Are pets permitted?

- If residents cannot bring their own furniture in, are the rooms well furnished and comfortable? Is there enough cupboard space, and somewhere to lock valuables away? Are the rooms in a good state of decoration and repair? Is there enough light and ventilation? Is there a good heating system which can be controlled in each room to individual preference?

- Can residents lock their rooms, so that they can have privacy when they want it? Is their privacy respected at all times?

- Is there a lift or stair-lift for people who can't manage stairs?
- Are there handrails on the stairs and in the corridors? Are there ramps for wheelchairs for small inclines?
- Can residents get up when they like, go to bed when they like, and have baths when they like, or are there regulations about this?
- Is there a varied menu and a balanced diet? Does the home cater for special diets (ie vegetarian, special religious requirements)? (You might ask to see the menus for a week, and to stay for a meal in order to try the food and service.) Are mealtimes flexible or rigid? Is breakfast served in residents' rooms, and are there facilities for them to make a cup of tea if they want one?
- Are the communal rooms – the lounge and dining-room – large and pleasant, and well furnished?
- Is there a television set on in the communal lounge, or are residents encouraged to have their own TV sets in their rooms, leaving the lounge peaceful and quiet for reading, a game of cards, or conversation? Is there a separate sitting-room for visitors?
- Are residents encouraged to do chores if they want to? Can they look after their own rooms, for instance?
- Are outings and social events organised for residents, and are they encouraged to take an interest in the running of the home – through a Residents' Committee, perhaps?
- Are residents encouraged to take up or continue favourite hobbies, such as gardening, or to attend classes and follow educational interests?
- Is there a visiting hairdresser, chiropodist, and physiotherapist?
- Can residents entertain visitors in their own rooms, and if not, is there a separate room where they can see visitors in private? Is there a guest room where visitors can stay overnight?

- Can residents retain the services of their own GPs, or are they expected to be looked after by the one doctor who visits the home?
- How many staff are there, and what is the ratio of staff to residents? What is the ratio of trained to untrained staff in a nursing home?
- How do staff address residents? Is their manner courteous and helpful? (You should observe the behaviour of the staff towards the residents.)
- What arrangements are there for any regular medication residents may need? Are they encouraged to keep and administer their own drugs, or are medicines kept in a safe place by the manager or matron, and handed out at regular intervals (say after meals)? If the latter, is a careful record kept of the dosages and the times when they are given?
- Will the home allow residents to stay if and when they become very frail, or will they have to move to other accommodation?
- How does the home present its accounts to residents? Do they receive a proper statement regularly, with details of all the items charged?
- Does the home allow residents to retain their own pension books?
- What are the conditions under which a resident's stay may be terminated by either side?
- Is there a satisfactory complaints procedure, and are complaints taken seriously and handled in a satisfactory way?
- Is the home of a size which is congenial to you: not too small, with residents living 'on top of one another', and not too large and impersonal?
- Can you communicate adequately if your first language is not English?

There are probably many other things you will want to know about the homes you are visiting and considering, but this is a basic list of questions which should help you to find out just how good a home is, and whether or not you would like to live in it. You can add to the list other points which occur to you.

The governing factor

There is one all-important, governing factor which affects the way every home is run, and that is the whole manner, personality, and approach of the person in charge. A home may be modest in the services and accommodation it provides, but if the owner/manager is wholly committed to the welfare of the residents, and has their well-being and happiness always at heart, it will be a contented and well-run place. But even the most luxurious, expensive home will be cold and uninviting if the person in charge lacks the special caring qualities needed for this job.

You can usually tell from the intangible atmosphere of a home, as well as from the attitude of the staff and the behaviour of the residents, whether or not the head of home has the right qualities and is of the calibre to do this responsible job. He or she must really care about the residents, be totally committed to their welfare, and have the quality of leadership which will imbue the rest of the staff with the same attitude. This is something you can only judge by your own instinctive reactions when you meet the head of home, and by your assessment of his or her personality, but it will be vitally important to your future happiness.

Chapter nine

How much will it cost, and how can I pay for it?

For most people the cost of going into a home, and how they will manage to pay the charges involved, is bound to be one of the most important factors they have to consider. How much you can afford to pay will inevitably govern your choice of home, so you will need to know not only the fees charged by different types of home but also what financial assistance you may be entitled to claim to supplement your own resources.

Local authority homes

Old people's homes provided by local authorities are intended for those living locally who are frail or disabled and in need of care and support which they cannot otherwise get. Many people living in these homes are subsidised by the local authority, and priority for places in them is naturally given to those in greatest need. It is not always realised that local authorities are obliged by law to assess people's incomes, and to levy charges according to a scale based on available income.

Each local authority fixes a standard weekly charge for its homes which is based on the actual running costs. Applicants for places are assessed for their ability to pay this standard charge, and those who cannot afford it will be offered a lower rate, based on their resources – both income and capital. There is a national minimum rate, which is based on the basic retirement pension plus an allowance for 'pocket money'.

The standard charge for the home would be considerably more than this: the present weekly charge (as of November 1987) in East Sussex, for example, is £136.78, which is fairly typical, although rates do of course vary round the country. This standard charge is also regarded as a maximum rate; that is to say, no resident would be expected to pay more than this.

If you decide to apply for a place in a local authority home, the social workers will need full details of your income and savings, and of any other assets you may have, such as property, so that they can work out how much you can afford to pay. You may, for instance, have a pension from your former job as well as your State pension; you may have put your savings into National Savings Certificates or a building society; and you may be the owner, or the joint owner, of the house in which you live. All these things will be taken into account by the local authority social services staff whose job it is to work out how much you can afford to pay towards your keep between the minimum and the maximum rates.

Your financial position

You will be given a Form of Financial Statement to fill in with all these details, and you will have to sign a declaration that all the information you have given is true and complete. If, incidentally, your State pension is less than the basic retirement pension, and you cannot afford to pay even the minimum charge, you can claim income support to bring it up to that level – provided, of course, that you do not have savings amounting to more than £6,000. No one with savings over that figure can claim income support.

If you live with your husband or wife, or other close relative, he or she will also have to fill in a similar form so that his or her financial circumstances are taken into account as well. Your spouse may be expected to contribute towards your upkeep in a local authority residential home, if he or she can afford to do so.

If you own your own home, its current market value will be assessed, and an 'assumed' weekly income figure will be based on this sum. This is not done in an arbitrary way; the DHSS has published a table for calculating income from capital in a Memorandum of Guidance for charging and assessment procedures to be used by all local authorities. The principle behind it is that since this type of accommodation is subsidised by the ratepayers, residents should be expected to draw on their capital assets as well as their income in order to pay for it, which seems fair enough.

If you have been living with a spouse, a relative, or in some instances a private carer, and they want to continue living in your home after you move out, the value of the house will probably not be taken as part of your capital assets at all. You should find out what the practice is in your own local authority.

Millicent Reynolds lived in a council flat on her own until her arthritis got so bad she couldn't manage any longer. She had had one hip replacement operation, but her knees were now affected, and her hands too were getting very stiff and deformed. She had worked as a shop assistant all her life, and had enjoyed the variety of being able to move from job to job, but she had no pension other than her State retirement pension. She had, however, managed to save £4,000, with which she had bought National Savings Certificates, and her younger brother sent her £6 a week, since she could not claim supplementary pension because of her savings. She was grateful for this extra money, as she found it difficult to manage on her State pension, especially in winter when her heating bills were large.

Millicent's GP wrote to the local social services department on her behalf recommending her for a place in residential care, and a social worker visited her to talk about this possibility, and to find out what her financial circumstances were. Eventually she was offered a place in a large but pleasant home nearby where the standard weekly charge was £100. Millicent was asked to pay £48.90 a week. This charge was based on her State retirement pension of £41.15 a week, plus £2 of the £6 from her brother, plus £14 a week from her savings, but deducting £8.25 a week as her personal allowance. The income from her savings was assessed at a rate of 25p for every £50, but the first £1,200 of her capital sum was 'disregarded' under the regulations laid down in the Memorandum of Guidance; the total taken into account was therefore £2,800. In the same way, £4 of the weekly £6 Millicent got from her brother was 'disregarded'. (NB figures are based on calculations from the state pension at 1988 rates.)

Private homes

The fees charged by privately owned homes can vary enormously, according to the type and quality of the accommodation offered. A modest home may charge in the region of £130 a week, while a luxurious one may charge up to £500 a week. 'You pays your money', as the saying goes, 'and you takes your choice'. But since it has been the policy of the DHSS that older people should not be kept in hospital but should be discharged home or to a residential home or nursing home as soon as possible, the DHSS will subsidise the cost of this through income support payments. A few health authorities also pay for beds in private nursing homes to which patients can be discharged from hospital if they need continued nursing care, but this is the exception rather than the rule.

Help from the DHSS

The same rule applies as to all income support: ie you cannot claim unless your savings amount to less than £6,000. If you are eligible to claim income support, however, you should contact the DHSS office in the area where the home you are moving to is situated, and they will send or give you the right form to fill in with details of your financial position. From this they will work out how much you can afford to pay towards the weekly charge; they will make up the difference, up to a limit which has been set by the DHSS, also allowing you an additional sum for personal expenses.

If you own a house, you will be expected to sell it in order to use the capital sum to pay for your nursing home or rest home place. Once it is clear that the stay in the home will be permanent you will be expected to raise the money to pay the home's fees through a loan or some other means while the sale of the house is going through. If you do not sell your home, its value will be taken into account as part of your capital, less the value of the mortgage, and 10 per cent to represent the notional costs of a sale. If your husband, wife, cohabitee, or other relative who is aged or incapacitated, continues to live in the house, however, it will not have to be sold.

If you are currently claiming Attendance Allowance, this will be taken fully into account when you are being assessed for benefit.

The limits laid down for weekly fees for residential and nursing care for elderly people were as follows in 1988:

Residential care homes for the elderly	£130	(London £147.50)
Residential care homes for the very dependent or blind elderly	£155	(London £172.50)

Nursing homes for the elderly	£185	(London £202.50)
Nursing homes for the mentally handicapped	£200	(London £217.50)
Nursing homes for the terminally ill	£230	(London £247.50)
Nursing homes for physical disability before pension age	£230	(London £247.50)

You will see that the fees increase according to the amount of care required, and that an extra allowance is made for homes in the London area, which is acknowledged to be more expensive.

Help from other sources

If the home you have decided to move into charges more than this, and you cannot afford to pay the extra, you may be able to get further help from a charity or benevolent fund. It is worth consulting such organisations as Counsel and Care for the Elderly, the Association of Charity Officers, or your local Citizens Advice Bureau. *The Charities Digest*, which should be in the reference section of your public library, also gives information about charitable organisations which might be helpful.

Malcolm Jackson, aged 78, was confused and aggressive in his behaviour, and when he began to lose his memory, and control of his personal habits, and also to wander the streets at all hours of the day and night when he could escape from his home, his wife asked their family doctor for more help, as she just couldn't cope any longer, being elderly herself. Their doctor called in a psychogeriatrician – a specialist who is expert in the mental disorders that afflict older people – who diagnosed dementia, and admitted Malcolm to hospital for treatment. Unfortunately, although his behaviour could be controlled by drugs, his condition would never improve, his wife was told, but would gradually get worse. It was not possible to keep Malcolm in hospital for the rest of his life, so the consultant psychogeriatrician recommended that he go into a nursing home which specialised in caring for mentally frail elderly people, and gave Malcolm's wife the address of one he knew was very good and conveniently placed for her. It was owned and managed by a psychiatric nurse (one with special training in nursing the mentally ill) and his wife, who was also a Registered Nurse. Both had trained and worked in the National Health Service before deciding to set up their own nursing home. The fees of the nursing home were £212 a week, towards which Malcolm could claim the nursing home limit for an elderly patient who is mentally ill (£185) plus his allowance of £9.55 for personal spending. His income, as assessed by social services department, was composed of his State pension, the higher attendance allowance, and income support, to make up the £185 a week limit. There was still over £25 a week to find, and as Malcolm had been a professional musician before he retired, his wife applied to the Musician's Benevolent Fund to see if they would help her. Fortunately they agreed to pay the extra to make up the nursing home's fees; Malcolm moved in, and his wife was able to visit him regularly to see that he was well cared for, and as comfortable as possible. (NB figures are current at 1988 levels.)

Voluntary homes

You can claim income support towards the cost of a place in a home run by a charitable or voluntary organisation in just the same way as for a private home. You would in any case have to fulfil whatever conditions the organisation had for admitting residents to one of its homes, and these of course vary from organisation to organisation. Their charges are unlikely to be exorbitant, by virtue of the fact that they are non-profit-making, but they do have to cover their costs and expenditure on maintenance and repairs.

Counting the cost

The cost of going into a home should not be a major obstacle, since the State is prepared to help its older people financially who need this refuge at the end of their lives. There is the benefit of knowing that all your living expenses – rates, heating, light, bed and board – will be taken care of, and all you will need money for is clothing, postage and phone calls, notepaper, personal needs such as soap and other toilet effects, gifts to friends and relatives, materials for hobbies (ie knitting wool, watercolour paints and brushes), drinks and confectionery, and other small items. The personal allowance permitted by the DHSS and the local authority may seem small, but some residents are apparently able to save a little: in East Sussex there is a banking system for residents in local authority homes who have their own personal accounts with the head of home, drawing out what they need and saving and investing the rest, so that they can accumulate a small lump sum to fall back on if and when they need it.

You will probably ask yourself now how you should choose between a local authority home, a private home, and a home owned and run by a charitable organisation. Broadly speaking, the difference is that local authorities are bound by law to provide residential care for the elderly who have become so frail they can no longer live in their own homes, and whose means are slender; while privately owned homes are commercial ventures – the proprietors must make a profit in order to be able to exist themselves. Voluntary or charitable homes come between the two: they are run by a wide variety of organisations as a service to particular professions, trades, religious faiths, or other groups of people of one kind or another, on a non-profit-making basis. Their charges are usually reasonable (although they may be expensive) because they are largely financed by donations and fund-raising, and any surplus is usually ploughed back into improving and developing their homes.

Priority for places in local authority homes rightly goes to those in greatest need of both financial and physical support, and if there is a long waiting list for vacancies an applicant might be told to look for private accommodation if his or her needs were not as great as those of other applicants. If that person could not afford the full charge, the local authority concerned might make up the difference.

Age Concern England produces two factsheets which may be useful: No. 10, "Local Authorities and Residential Care", and No. 11, "Income Support for Residential Homes and Nursing Care". They are free on receipt of a stamped, addressed envelope.

Chapter ten

What will it be like, and how will I cope?

There's no avoiding the fact that moving into a home after a lifetime of freedom and independence is a major upheaval which can present problems. However carefully you and your relatives have tried to make sure the home you have chosen is the kind of place where you can be happy, you will have to adapt yourself to a new way of life which at first may seem strange and even unwelcome. Instead of being your own master in your own home, you will be living in an establishment geared to the needs of the residents, and therefore with certain rules and regulations. You will be dependent on others for most of the essentials of daily living, such as meals and laundry, and possibly also washing and dressing yourself if you are handicapped by a disease such as arthritis. You will be living cheek by jowl with people whom you may not necessarily like, or whose personal habits irritate you, or whose behaviour is disruptive. You will have to depend on staff whose way of doing things is not necessarily your way.

Peace of mind

On the plus side, however, once you have settled in, you will find enormous relief at the fact that you don't have to worry any longer about the everyday tasks of cooking, shopping, housework, and gardening, which become more and more difficult and time-consuming with age. You won't have to worry so much about your own safety – about possible falls when there is no one to come to your assistance, or accidents in a part of your home where you can't call for help or make the neighbours hear you. You won't have to worry about falling ill: there will always be someone at hand whose job it is to look after you and give you all the help you need. You will gain a great sense of security, though you will still want to control your own life.

The secret of settling happily into your 'home from home' seems to lie, first, in making the decision to go there on your own, and not allowing yourself to be persuaded into it by some well-meaning friend or relative, possibly against your better judgment. You must be absolutely sure in your own mind that this is the only way forward for you. You must weigh up all the pros and cons very carefully, looking at the disadvantages as well as the advantages calmly and objectively, so that when you have made your decision you will know that you will only have yourself to blame if it doesn't work out well. There is nothing worse than finding yourself in an unhappy situation because you have been pressurised or forced into it by others against your will or better judgment. You will blame the person who persuaded you, you will be filled with resentment and anger as well as unhappiness, and you will never be able to come to terms with or adapt to your new existence. So, first and foremost, make your own decision. Then, oddly enough, you will find it much easier to take any problems or difficulties in your stride.

Second, be philosophic; accept the fact that in order to gain something, one usually has to give something else up – in this case, you have to give up a measure of freedom and independence in exchange for security and support. Once you have accepted this fact of life, it will be easier to take what comes and meet people in your new surroundings half way.

Someone else's experience

Let three old people, all in their eighties, who have gone through this experience give you their advice.

First let's meet Mrs Hayhoe, who has been a resident in a voluntary home for five years. She is a widow who, she says, made the great mistake after her husband died of moving away from her home town in Surrey to be near her son in the Midlands. She felt an unwelcome foreigner in her new surroundings – a bungalow on a council estate – and when her son changed his job and moved away from the district, she was lonely and utterly miserable. 'Older people should never move away from their homes to be near their family', she says.

Eventually she became ill and knew the time had come to go into a home, although her daughter thought she wasn't the type to settle in easily. On the first day in her new 'home from home' she was so unhappy she could have run away. However, she made up her mind to try and be contented for the sake of her children. She stuck it out, and now, five years later, she is happily settled and enjoys life. What Mrs Hayhoe found most difficult to adapt to, after a lifetime of being 'boss' of her own family, in her own house, was losing that authority and independence. She took badly to life in an institution (for that is what any home for elderly people, large or small, is bound to be) where she was subject to rules and regulations, and dependent on others for her daily needs. She would have liked to do things for herself and other people. But once she had accepted this, she found it was a great relief not to have to worry about such chores as shopping or cooking, and was able to enjoy the new freedom that this gave her. 'It makes all the difference having a room of your own, though', she says.

Second, meet Miss Ivy Brereton, a lively, active, single lady of 87, who moved into the same home just eight weeks ago. She had worked all her life, and lived with and looked after her mother, who died at the age of 94. When she began to feel the need of care herself, Miss Brereton moved into a privately owned rest home, where to begin with she was happy and comfortable. The home changed hands, however, and the new management was not nearly so good, so after looking around for a while Miss Brereton found a 'sheltered' flat in a block supervised by a warden, where she was extremely happy and well looked after. At last, though, after a series of illnesses, operations, and accidents – a hip replacement, a cataract removal, developing Paget's disease of bone, fracturing first a leg, and then four ribs in a nasty fall at home – she decided enough was enough and found herself a room in a combined residential care and nursing home run by a professional Benevolent Fund, to which she had subscribed.

Miss Brereton has taken a positive, practical approach to this important move, not allowing sentiment to influence her in getting rid of her furniture and possessions – 'I have never been tied to possessions, and my nephews and nieces were very glad to have what I gave them' – or regret to discolour her view of her new life in the home. 'While you can live independently try to go on doing so, because it does you good to have to get out and shop and to cook for yourself, and make all the other efforts required to look after yourself. But when you see the signs that you are soon going to need help, don't wait to start planning and looking around for the right sort of accommodation. Then you won't be taken unprepared by events, but be able to choose carefully among the options open to you.'

Miss Brereton puts her success at adapting to her new life down to temperament, to the fact that she has always accepted responsibility for her own life and made her own decisions, and that she has chosen a home which is in the town where she has lived for years and where she has many friends. She had already joined the Women's Institute and various other clubs and societies, so has been able to keep up her interests and hobbies.

She enjoys reading and spends a little time every day reading to one of her fellow residents, who is blind. She makes a point of being sociable with other residents, but at the same time enjoys the privacy of her own room, as well as outings arranged by the clubs and associations to which she belongs.

Finally, may I introduce you to Mr Kirkham, aged 86 ('I'm one of the youngsters round here'), who is a widower, diabetic and deaf, and has lived in the home for nine months. When his wife became seriously ill he moved with her to a flat near his son and daughter-in-law, on the advice of his doctor. After she died he was able to carry on living on his own for some years, with home help and meals-on-wheels, and regular weekend visits to his son. But things got more and more difficult for him, and one day he said to his son: 'I've had enough, I don't want to stop here any longer.' A family conference was held with his daughter flying over from America, and it was decided to find him a place in a home, where he could take one or two treasured possessions with him.

On the day he moved in, and watched his family driving away, he felt very shaky, and asked himself whether he would ever see them or his friends again. Up to then he had always slept in the big double bed he and his wife had shared, and more than anything else he found it upsetting to have to sleep in a narrow single bed. 'It's small things like that which can be difficult', he says. But gradually, and with perseverance on his part, he became accustomed to his new life, and began to feel at home in his 'home from home'. He appreciates the excellent medical and nursing care he is given for his diabetes, and having his treasured armchair and bureau in his room makes all the difference. He has made good friends with other residents and with staff in the home.

'You have to be patient and philosophical, be prepared to accept anything that comes along, and to make the best of things, and gradually you will begin to feel at home', he says. 'We only go through this life once, after all.' Mr Kirkham is a

Christian, which has helped him greatly, and he believes that religious faith of any kind is a great support at this time of life.

Miss Brereton echoes his thoughts. Her advice to readers is: 'Try to look for the good things, don't look for what is wrong. Things may not be done your way, but that doesn't mean it is not the right way.' All three were critical of fellow residents who were perpetual 'moaners', complaining about everything all the time. They firmly believed that it is up to each individual to try to make a success of this new life. As Miss Brereton trenchantly said: 'You take yourself with you wherever you go.'

A home from home

Four important points emerged from these conversations to help you as you begin your search for a 'home from home'.

First, unless you particularly want to share a room with your spouse or a close friend, it is very important to have your own room where you can enjoy privacy when you want to, and keep a few of your cherished possessions around you. Remember that you will be surrounded by other people in the home all the time, some of whom may be difficult in their habits and behaviour because of their age and disabilities, so it will be easier for you to tolerate them if you can retreat to the peace and quiet of your own room occasionally. It is also important to have a toilet within easy reach of your room, though even better to have one of your own: some new homes are being designed with each room having its own toilet and washing facilities, which is ideal.

Second, try to find a home which is not only well managed but also where there will be continuity of management. The quality of life in a home will be governed by the person in charge, but even though you find one that seems really good, remember that if it changes hands its standards could deteriorate sharply under the new management. Miss Brereton went through this experience, and suggests that a home owned by a large organisation, possibly a charitable body of some kind, is most likely to set and maintain good standards and employ staff of high quality.

Third, don't move away from your home locality to be near your son or daughter unless you know and like the district where they live, and are as certain as you can be that they won't move away. Remember that people do change their jobs, or decide to go abroad, and that marriages do break down. If you stay in your home town or district, where you have good friends and neighbours and belong to active clubs and societies, you will still be in your familiar surroundings and able to continue to enjoy your leisure interests and social life. Also you won't feel that you are a burden to your family in any way.

Fourth, final, and most important: no one but you can make a success of your new life once you have taken the plunge and moved in. It will be a big change in your life and one that will require a lot of effort to adapt to, but if you accept this and look for the positive benefits rather than the negative drawbacks, the best rather than the worst, you will gradually settle into your new life and realise that you have indeed found a 'home from home'.

Booklist

Health

Better Health in Retirement by J A Muir Gray,
   Age Concern England, 1982, £1.20

Age and Vitality by Irene Gore,
   Age Concern England, £1.30

Eating Well on a Budget
   BBC Food and Drink Programme and Age Concern England, 1987, £1.50

Eat Well, Stay Well – Healthy Eating for People over 60 and
Eat Well, Stay Well for Afro-Caribbean Pensioners
   Age Concern Greater London, 50p each

Cooking Made Easy for Disabled People by Audrey Ellis,
   Sainsbury's Food Guide

Balancing Your Diet – How to Eat Sensibly and Well
by Jenny Salmon,
   Sainsbury's Food Guide

Know Your Medicines by Pat Blair,
   Age Concern England, 1985, £3.75

Caring for a relative

Nursing the Aged by Pat Young,
  Woodhead Faulkner Ltd, 1984

Caring for Elderly People – Understanding and Practical Help by Susan Hooker,
  Routledge and Kegan Paul, 1981

Caring for an Elderly Relative by Dr Keith Thompson,
  Martin Dunitz, 1986

Taking Care of your Elderly Relative by Dr J A Muir Gray and Heather MacKenzie,
  Penguin, 1986

The 36-Hour Day: *Caring at Home for Confused Elderly People* by Mace, Rabins, Cloke and McEwen,
  Age Concern England, 1985, £6.95

General books

Survival Guide for Widows by June Hemer and Ann Stanyer,
  Age Concern England, 1986, £3.50

What Every Woman Should Know About Retirement, edited by Helen Franks,
  Age Concern England, 1987, £4.50

Housing

Owning Your Home in Retirement by David Bookbinder,
  Age Concern England and the National Housing and

Town Planning Council, available from Age Concern England, 1987, £1.50

Housing Options for Older People by David Bookbinder, Age Concern England, 1987, £2.50

A Buyer's Guide to Sheltered Housing Age Concern England, 1986, £1.00

Finance

Your Rights: A Guide to Benefits for Retired People
Annual publication from Age Concern England, 90p

Your Taxes and Savings in Retirement
Annual publication from Age Concern England, £2.50

Residential care

Home Life: A Code of Practice for Residential Care
 Centre for Policy on Ageing, 1983, £3.30 available from Bailey Bros, Warner House, Folkestone, Kent CT19 6PH

Registration and Inspection of Nursing Homes: A Handbook for Health Authorities,
 National Association of Health Authorities in England and Wales, 1985. NAHA, Garth House, 47 Edgbaston Park Road, Birmingham B15 2RS

Croner's Care Homes Guide (2 vols by region)
 Croner Publications Ltd.

Charities Digest, annual publication
 from the Family Welfare Association.

Directory of Private Hospitals and Health Services,
published by Longmans

All Age Concern publications are available from the following address:
Marketing Department,
60 Pitcairn Road,
Mitcham, Surrey, CR4 3LL.
Price includes postage and packing.

National Organisations that may help

Asian Sheltered Residential Accommodation (ASRA)
5a Westminster Bridge Road
London SE1 7XW
Tel: 01-928 8108 ext 40

Abbeyfield Society
186/192 Darkes Lane
Potters Bar
Herts EN6 1AB
Tel: 0707 44845

Age Concern England
Bernard Sunley House
60 Pitcairn Road
Mitcham
Surrey CR4 3LL
Tel: 01-640 5431

Age Concern Scotland
33 Castle Street
Edinburgh EH2 3DN
Tel: 031-225 5000

Age Concern Wales
1 Cathedral Road
Cardiff CF1 9SD
Tel: 0222 371566
or 371821

Age Concern Northern Ireland
6 Lower Crescent
Belfast BT7 1NR
Tel: 0232 245729

Anchor Housing Assoc.
13-15 Magdalen Street
Oxford OX1 3BP
Tel: 0865 722261

Arthritis Care
6 Grosvenor Crescent
London SW1X 7ER
Tel: 01-235 0902

Arthritis and Rheumatism Council
41 Eagle Street
London WC1R 4AR
Tel: 01-405 8572

NATIONAL ORGANISATIONS THAT MAY HELP

Association of Carers
21-23 New Road
Chatham
Kent ME4 4QJ
Tel: 0634 813981

Association of Charity Officers
c/o Royal Institute of Chartered Surveyors (RICS) Benevolent Fund Ltd
2nd Floor
Tavistock House North
Tavistock Square
London WC1H 9RJ
Tel: 01-387 0578

British Federation of Care Home Proprietors
51 Leopold Road
Felixstowe
Suffolk IP11 7NR
Tel: 0394 279539

Cancer Relief/MacMillan Fund
see National Society for Cancer Relief

Central Council for Jewish Social Services
212 Golders Green Road
London NW11 9DW
Tel: 01-458 3282

Chest, Heart and Stroke Association
Tavistock House North
Tavistock Square
London WC1H 9JE
Tel: 01-387 3012

Court of Protection
Stewart House
24 Kingsway
London WC2B 6HD
Tel: 01-405 4300

Counsel and Care for the Elderly
131 Middlesex Street
London E1 7JF
Tel: 01-621 1624

College of Health *(part of the Consumers' Association)*
2 Marylebone Road
London NW1 4DX
Tel: 01-935 2460

Cruse
Cruse House
126 Sheen Road
Richmond
Surrey TW9 1UR
Tel: 01-940 4818

Department of Health and Social Security (DHSS)
Alexander Fleming Hse.
Elephant & Castle
London SE1 6BY
Tel: 01-407 5522

NATIONAL ORGANISATIONS THAT MAY HELP

Disability Alliance
25 Denmark Street
London WC2H 8NJ
Tel: 01-240 0806

Disabled Living Foundation
380/384 Harrow Road
London W9 2HU
Tel: 01-289 6111

Elderly Accommodation Counsel Ltd.
1 Durward House
31 Kensington Court
London W8 5BH
Tel: 01-937 8709

English National Board of Nursing, Midwifery and Health Visiting
170 Tottenham Court Road
London W1P OHA
Tel: 01-388 3131

General Medical Council
44 Hallam Street
London W1N 6AE
Tel: 01-580 7642

GRACE *(Gould's Residential Advisory Centre for the Elderly)*
PO Box 71
Cobham
Surrey KT11 2JR
Tel: 01-0932 62928/65765

The Health Service Commissioner (Ombudsman)
Church House
Great Smith Street
London SW1P 3BW
Tel: 01-212 7676

Jewish Welfare Board
221 Golders Green Road
London NW11 9DW
Tel: 01-458 3282

Keep Fit Association
16 Upper Woburn Place
London WC1H OQG
Tel: 01-387 4349

MacMillan Nursing Service
(c/o National Society for Cancer Relief)

Marie Curie Memorial Foundation
28 Belgrave Square
London SW1X 8QG
Tel: 01-235 3325

MIND *(National Association for Mental Health)*
22 Harley Street
London W1N 2ED
Tel: 01-637 0741

120 NATIONAL ORGANISATIONS THAT MAY HELP

National Association for Widows
Neville House
14 Waterloo Street
Birmingham B2 5UG
Tel: 021-643 8348
(10.00 am to 4.00 pm Monday to Friday)

National Council for Carers and their Elderly Dependants
29 Chilworth Mews
London W2 3RG
Tel: 01-724 7776

National Confederation of Registered Residential Care Homes Association (NCRRHA)
8 Southampton Place
London WC1A 2EF
Tel: 01-405 2277

National Society for Cancer Relief
Anchor House
15-19 Britten Street
London SW3 3TZ
Tel: 01-351 7811

RADAR *(Royal Association for Disability and Rehabilitation)*
25 Mortimer Street
London W1N 8AB
Tel: 01-637 5400

Registered Nursing Home Association
Calthorpe House
Hagley Road
Edgbaston
Birmingham B16 8QY
Tel: 021-454 2511

SCEMSC *(Standing Conference of Ethnic Minority Senior Citizens)*
5-5a Westminster Bridge Road
London SE1 7XW
Tel: 01-928 0095

Scottish National Board for Nursing, Midwifery and Health Visiting
22 Queen Street
Edinburgh EH2 1SX
Tel: 031 226 7371

UK Central Council for Nursing, Midwifery and Health Visiting
23 Portland Place
London W1N 3AF
Tel: 01-637 7181

Welsh National Board for Nursing, Midwifery and Health Visiting
Pearl Assurance House
Greyfriars Road
Cardiff CF1 3AG
Tel: 0222 395535